LISTENING, LEARNING, CARING & COUNSELLING

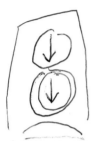

Dr Cate Howell is a GP and therapist, researcher, lecturer and author. She has over 30 years of training and experience in the health area, with a special interest in mental health and assisting individuals experiencing life stresses or crises. Cate holds a Bachelor in Applied Science (Occupational Therapy), a Bachelor of Medicine, a Bachelor of Surgery, a Masters in Health Service Management and a Doctor of Philosophy (Medicine). She also has a Diploma in Clinical Hypnosis and has trained in Couple Therapy, Cognitive Behavioural Therapy (CBT), Acceptance and Commitment Therapy (ACT) and Interpersonal Therapy (IPT). She has travelled internationally to present research findings on depression and has been published in a number of academic journals. The author of three books, Cate was awarded the Order of Australia Medal in 2012 for services to medicine, particularly mental health, and professional organizations.

LISTENING, LEARNING, CARING & COUNSELLING

The Essential Manual for Psychologists, Psychiatrists, Counsellors & Other Healthcare Professionals on Caring for Their Clients

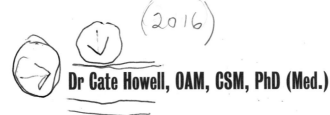

Dr Cate Howell, OAM, CSM, PhD (Med.)

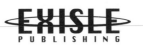
EXISLE
PUBLISHING

First published 2016

Exisle Publishing Pty Ltd
'Moonrising', Narone Creek Road, Wollombi, NSW 2325, Australia
P.O. Box 60–490, Titirangi, Auckland 0642, New Zealand
www.exislepublishing.com

A CiP record for this book is available from the National Library of Australia.

ISBN 978-1-925335-04-0

Designed by Nick Turzynski, redinc. Book Design
Typeset in Baskerville 10/15
Printed in China

This book uses paper sourced under ISO 14001 guidelines from well-managed forests and other
controlled sources.

10 9 8 7 6 5 4 3 2 1

Disclaimer

This book is a general guide only and should never be a substitute for the skill, knowledge and
experience of a qualified medical professional dealing with the facts, circumstances and symptoms
of a particular case. The nutritional, medical and health information presented in this book is
based on the research, training and professional experience of the author, and is true and complete
to the best of their knowledge. However, this book is intended only as an informative guide; it
is not intended to replace or countermand the advice given by the reader's personal physician.
Because each person and situation is unique, the author and the publisher urge the reader to
check with a qualified healthcare professional before using any procedure where there is a question
as to its appropriateness. The author, publisher and their distributors are not responsible for
any adverse effects or consequences resulting from the use of the information in this book. It is
the responsibility of the reader to consult a physician or other qualified healthcare professional
regarding their personal care. This book contains references to products that may not be available
everywhere. The intent of the information provided is to be helpful; however, there is no guarantee
of results associated with the information provided.

This book is dedicated to Alex and to two good friends, Meredith and Michele. It is dedicated to past teachers, and especially the clients I have travelled with, as they have taught me so much. I thank you.

CONTENTS

Introduction

At the centre of any caring role is listening attentively to the concerns, stories and needs of others. Whether you are a counsellor, health professional or therapist, you are essentially a guide and educator for the clients or patients with whom you work, to facilitate their learning and recovery. This work will also, no doubt, ignite a passion for ongoing learning. You can choose to learn through reading, self-reflection, studying online, attending courses for professional development or undertaking supervision. You also learn a great deal from your colleagues but most importantly from your clients, and you will learn a lot about yourself in the process. At the heart of the approach in *Listening, Learning, Caring & Counselling* — known more simply as LLCC — is *caring* or kindness, and you care for your clients in different capacities. You may have chosen to specifically counsel, or you might find it is an important aspect of your work although not the main focus.

If you are, or are training to be, a counsellor, mental health professional (such as a psychologist or social worker, a medical practitioner, psychiatrist, mental health nurse or nurse practitioner), allied health professional (physiotherapist, occupational therapist, dietician), psychotherapist, crisis or school counsellor, then different aspects of LLCC will have relevance for you. The LLCC approach aims to be a guide, full of ideas, and to become an essential and faithful companion to you in your work. It will cover key fundamental areas, the 'bread and butter' of most practice. However, it cannot cover everything, and so more specialized areas such as addiction, pain and eating-related issues have not been included. In addition, the focus of LLCC is on adults.

You might also ask, why is a doctor writing about LLCC? I began my career as an occupational therapist working on oncology and cardiac units and later in the fields of rehabilitation and psychiatry. Occupational Therapy focuses on helping clients function in all areas of life, including the psychosocial, which became a passion for me. Later I decided to study medicine, training as a general practitioner (GP), again being drawn to the psychological aspects of medicine.

As a result, I pursued training in hypnotherapy, couple therapy and a range of other psychotherapies. I undertook a Churchill Fellowship studying the management of anxiety and depression, and a PhD in the area of depression followed. I worked at a university to help establish a program in counselling and psychotherapy, have written several books on mental health topics, and for many years now my practice has focused primarily on mental health and counselling. In 2012 I was awarded an Australia Day Honour, the Order of Australia Medal, for services to mental health. Over the years I have worked with thousands of clients and taught thousands of students, across Australia and internationally.

The aim of this book is to share existing knowledge in the field of caring and counselling as well as some of the experience I have gained throughout my career. This is not a book about fundamental counselling skills as there are several very good books already available on this, and these will be referred to in the first few chapters. However, I review a few of the important concepts in relation to communication and relating to clients; then the main emphasis is on how to assist clients as they work through the issues they commonly face, such as low mood, relationship issues or loss and grief. In addressing these issues, I draw primarily from a range of established and *evidence-based* principles and therapies.

The focus of this book is on adults; it is **not** a book about fundamental counselling skills but focuses on practical applications.

Practitioners may specialize in one therapy. However, over my years of working as a doctor and therapist I have learnt to favour an *integrative approach*, utilizing a range of approaches and therapies to assist the person, depending on the individual and the issues, as 'one size does not fit all'.[1] This metaphor can also be extended to health professionals and counsellors, as we are not all the same and our own personality and style will influence the approaches and therapies that we utilize. As a result, a number of different therapies and their related techniques will be described and incorporated into the LLCC approach, which will be explored in the first part of this book.

Above all, this book is a *practical* and user-friendly resource, with case studies (written as individual client stories), skills and tips for everyday practice.

The book is divided into three parts: Part 1: Foundations of the LLCC approach; Part 2: Managing life issues and problem areas; Part 3: Further LLCC key foundations.

Each part contains a number of chapters covering key topics. Part 2 is the largest and is the 'how to' part of the book. In terms of making the best use of this book, I recommend you take the following approach.

- Read Part 1 first as it provides foundation knowledge and introduces the integrative LLCC approach.
- Then read Part 2, or dip into the various chapters as you need to when addressing different issues with clients.
- Digest and refer to Part 3 as it contains vital information to be aware of to help you manage crises in practice, and to take care of yourself.

There are tools for you to use with clients both within the text and in the Appendix. When using these tools, the aim is for the client to complete them, with your guidance. So hand over the pen to the client wherever possible, and you may choose to give some of the tasks to the client as take-home tasks to do between sessions. This will depend on how motivated and focused the client is, so begin with small tasks when you think they are ready and build up as appropriate for the client.

Key points to remember are highlighted in boxes throughout the book. In addition, watch out for the 'LLCC tips'. These are ideas that have proved very helpful for clients, and you might like to incorporate them into your work. A client story is highlighted at the start of each chapter in Part 2 and referred to again later in the chapter as the LLCC management approach unfolds. Suggestions about how to incorporate Bibliotherapy and e-mental health are also included, and a range of resources are highlighted at the end of each chapter. Please also note that (not to take away from anyone's field of work, but simply to make wording less repetitious) the terms 'counsellor' and 'client' will be used in the text.

As mentioned earlier, at the heart of counselling and therapy is *caring*, and nothing must detract from this. Counselling and therapy approaches and skills build upon this to provide the means to educate, guide and help the client make shifts in their thinking or ways of being. Working in this field means that you are committed to life-long learning and growth. There is so much to learn and so many fascinating ideas to explore. I am very pleased that LLCC can be part of your journey.

So let's get started with the LLCC approach.

For blogs, meditation recordings and other information, please see my website: www.drcatehowell.com.au

1 FOUNDATIONS OF THE LLCC APPROACH

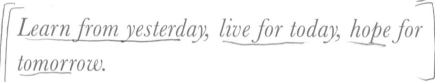

Learn from yesterday, live for today, hope for tomorrow.

—ALBERT EINSTEIN

There are some fundamental areas of knowledge, as well as key attitudes and skills, which underpin effective counselling. These foundations are relevant to any of the roles you might fulfil, and they include establishing a trusting relationship with your client and communicating effectively with them. The LLCC framework involves an integrative approach to counselling, and it includes making use of your clinical intuition skills. Comprehensive assessment is the basis of sound practice. **Part 1** outlines these very important foundations, whereas **Part 2** covers key issues of client concern and how these can be managed.

Chapter 1
The fundamentals of counselling

Perhaps one did not want to be loved so much as to be understood.

—**GEORGE ORWELL**

While all of the topics included in Part 1 are vital components of caring and counselling, the first fundamentals to establish are:

- definitions
- the therapeutic relationship
- effective communication
- the role of 'clinical intuition'
- the integrative approach
- consumer/carer perspectives
- cultural and gender issues.

Firstly, consider the following case study of Rosie, a counselling student on her first placement, and then as you read this chapter reflect on how the ideas presented might help her. You will hear more about Rosie later.

Rosie's story

Rosie did her undergraduate degree in Arts, and decided to do a postgraduate counselling course. She enjoyed all of the subjects in the first year, particularly the theory about counselling and learning how to listen to and empathize with people.

In the first two weeks of the placement, Rosie sat in and watched some sessions with clients. Then she started working with a couple of clients, but soon after reported that she was struggling to feel confident in herself and her ability to establish a good connection with her clients.

Definitions

Let's explore a few notions in relation to the definitions of caring, counselling and psychotherapy:

Caring refers to displaying kindness and concern for others, and is the practice of looking after those unable to care for themselves.[1]

Counselling and psychotherapy are professional activities that utilize an interpersonal relationship to enable people to develop self-understanding and to make changes in their lives.[2]

The counsellor is seen as a client's fellow traveller on road of life, not that different from the person who has come for help.[3]

Dr David Horgan, a Melbourne psychiatrist who focuses on depression treatment, describes psychotherapy as problem-sharing so that you are not alone in dealing with it, putting emotions into words, mastering thoughts and overcoming demoralization.[4]

For more information about definitions, refer to a number of excellent counselling texts, such as Corey, Egan, and Hutchinson.[5,6,7]

The therapeutic relationship

In the counselling process, the therapeutic relationship or connection with the client is the key to change and successful outcomes. Research suggests that the relationship between client and counsellor, and client factors are the main predictors of effective therapy.[8] A trusting and safe relationship forms the basis of the therapeutic relationship, which enables the client and therapist to work together towards understanding and change.

The first step is building a trusting connection or rapport, and a safe space to explore and share. I have heard many experts in the field say that the techniques used in counselling are secondary to the relationship itself, and I cannot agree more.

The therapeutic relationship with the client is the key to change and successful outcomes.

Humanistic psychology provides many interesting ideas that have influenced our thinking on the therapeutic relationship. This arm of psychology was pioneered by Abraham Maslow, who held the positive view that humans have natural potential. He studied 'self-actualizing' people and found they were self-aware, caring, trusting, creative and autonomous, in addition to being able to accept themselves and cope with uncertainty. Maslow decided that to self-actualize, humans needed to meet a range of needs, from basic physiological needs to belonging and love, and a need for esteem.[9] Carl Rogers, an academic and spokesperson for humanistic psychology, adopted this philosophy and developed 'person-centred therapy'. Rogers maintained that people have many resources within themselves and are capable of awareness and growth.[10]

Rogers identified three therapist attributes that create a growth-promoting environment:

- congruence (genuineness)
- unconditional positive regard (acceptance, caring)
- empathic understanding.[11]

He noted that these are central to developing a nurturing relationship and assisting the client. The therapeutic relationship involves feeling comfortable working together towards defined goals, and developing a sense of bonding. It involves being open, respectful and warm, and having the capacity to understand the client's view of themselves and the world.[12]

The therapeutic relationship is established through:

- creating a safe place
- explaining issues related to confidentiality, and adhering to them
- listening carefully
- being understanding and empathic
- establishing trust and respect
- being non-judgmental
- showing compassion
- seeing the client as the expert in their own life
- having a consistent approach, setting boundaries in the relationship
- effective communication.

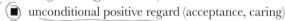

It is essential for the therapeutic relationship that the counsellor develops **self-awareness**. This may involve awareness of your own thoughts and feelings, and your relationships.[13] Counsellors often engage in their own counselling or psychotherapy to understand themselves more fully and to work through any issues. They must also be aware of the dynamics occurring within the therapeutic relationship. There is always a level of 'transference' and 'counter-transference' as counselling is a relationship. **Transference** refers to the client unconsciously projecting onto the counsellor positive or negative feelings from past relationships. An example would be projection of negative feelings such as mistrust, dependence or anger.[14] **Counter-transference** is defined as redirection of a counsellor's feelings towards a client, perhaps because they remind us of someone we have strong feelings about.[15] We may then experience emotions when working with a client, such as anger or jealousy, which have no relation to the client.

It is essential for the therapeutic relationship that the counsellor develops self-awareness . . . which involves self-reflection.

It is important to be aware of and manage these dynamics. If not, problems such as blurred boundaries, inappropriate disclosure of information or therapeutic breakdown can occur. It is therefore suggested to practise **self-reflection**. To aid understanding, you might ask yourself 'Am I responding in a way that feels like me? Do I associate this client with anyone else? What feelings do I have about them? Why am I feeling like this? How is it impacting on my work with this client?'[16] You may want to talk with a supervisor in relation to these aspects of working with the client.

Self-awareness also involves acknowledging your *values* in life and in relation to counselling. These influence how we act professionally. We need to consider that our values may differ from those of others, including our clients, but we need to respect other people's values. Consider your values as you read this section, and write them down where you can add to them or refer back to them later. They are very important, and to start you thinking, here are some examples cited in Hutchinson. Consider whether these values fit with yours, or whether other values guide you in your counselling work:

- We are all born with innate strengths and resources.
- The primary role of the counsellor is to help clients recognize their own capacity to make changes in their lives.

■ The driving force in counselling is caring and compassion.
■ Approach life with an attitude of gratitude and forgiveness.[17]

Take a few moments to reflect on and make a note of the values that drive you in your role as a counsellor. When you are feeling inspired, or worn out, or when you are looking for a change in role, it can be helpful to review these values.

Self-awareness . . . involves acknowledging your values in life and in relation to counselling.

Effective communication

Counselling essentially involves conversations between the client and counsellor, and it is through language and conversation that we create a sense of meaning and understanding in our lives. The importance of effective and empathic communication with the client cannot be emphasized enough. Some of the key communication skills will be touched on here.

It is through language and conversation that we create a sense of meaning and understanding in our lives.

When you first meet the client, it is essential to engage with them. This involves:
- welcoming the client and introducing yourself
- noticing non-verbal behaviours that give you information about how they are feeling, such as signs of nervousness or tension
- being aware of your own non-verbal behaviours (remember to sit squarely so you are facing the client, to have an open posture and to lean forward)
- finding a balance between self-awareness and not being preoccupied
- being interested and curious, utilizing questions at the outset
- being relaxed.[18]

Counselling employs a range of communication skills, and some of the essential ones include the following:

- Use prompts to show the client you are paying attention and to encourage them to tell you more, such as verbal prompts: 'mm hm', 'yes', uh huh', 'okay', 'I see'; or non-verbal, for example, leaning forward and back, gestures, nods and eye movements.
- Explore with a range of questions. These may be open ('How have you been feeling recently?', 'What has brought you to see me today?') to begin the conversation and to encourage further elaboration; or closed ('Do you know what she did then?', 'Does that concern you?') to elicit specific information.
- Listen actively, or pay attention fully. This is a vital skill in counselling, if not the most important skill to practise. Listen for both obvious and hidden content. To practise this skill you will need to be mindful and quieten your own thoughts.

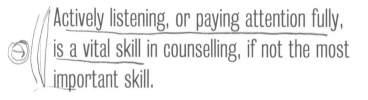

Actively listening, or paying attention fully, is a vital skill in counselling, if not the most important skill.

- Reflect the content and emotion of what the client is telling you, to assist them in understanding what has been happening in their life and to normalize and express their feelings.
  - Reflect content by paraphrasing or restating the most important part of what a client has said. These steps may assist:
    1. Recall the client's message and identify key content.
    2. Choose a beginning for your reflection, such as; 'It sounds like', 'So you think that' or 'It seems like'.
    2. Restate the content in your own words.
  - Reflect the client's feelings to let them know that you understand and are tuned in to their emotions. An example would be: 'It seems like you are feeling disappointed and distressed.'
  - Combine content and feeling reflections where appropriate: 'It seems like the recent disagreement with your colleague has really upset you, and that you are feeling quite down about the situation.'
- Utilize clarifying questions to help you understand the exact nature of what's been said by the client: 'And so you spoke with both your brother and sister about the events at the wedding, and they had the same understanding as you?' Clarification may involve reflecting what the

client has said, and then asking whether what you have said is correct: 'Is that how it is for you?'

- Summarize periodically in the conversation, as this emphasizes and ties together themes, can identify patterns and helps you both focus on important issues. This skill can be particularly useful at the start or end of a session, to review progress, or act as a transition when changing topics.
- Affirming and validating the client is important and powerful: 'You have been through a very difficult time, and shown a great deal of common sense and resilience in managing the challenges.'
- Remember to be yourself and develop your own style when incorporating these skills.

Affirming and validating the client is important and powerful.

Clinical intuition

The best and most beautiful things in the world cannot be seen or even touched. They must be felt with the heart.

—HELEN KELLER

You are probably familiar with intuition or 'knowing without knowing how you know', but you may not be so familiar with the term 'clinical intuition'. There is, in fact, more being written about this phenomenon in health and self-help literature as time goes on. Counselling texts now speak of listening for the unspoken in counselling as a meditative and intuitive process.[19] A useful definition of clinical intuition is that it 'involves sensing what is happening behind the client's words and beyond conscious awareness'.[20] Hutchinson refers to expressing your hunches about what is below the surface as 'wondering out loud', leading you to ask questions such as 'I wonder what the issue is?' or 'I wonder what would happen if . . .?'[21]

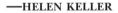

This growing interest in the role of intuition in therapy has occurred partly because of recent neurobiology findings, highlighting the role of the unconscious mind in 'clinical intuition'. Experienced counsellors utilize implicit knowledge that is housed in the non-dominant brain. Both the brain's left and right hemispheres have a range of roles. There is overlap in functions but, in general, if you are right-handed, the left or 'dominant' hemisphere houses the verbal and non-intuitive functions of the brain, whereas the right brain is the site of the visual, creative and intuitive functions.[22] Intuition is seen as potentially filling the gap between theory and practice. A number of authors agree that clinical intuition is necessary to facilitate deep change during counselling.[23]

Clinical intuition involves 'listening for the unspoken' and it 'fills the gap between theory and practice'.

Marks-Tarlow, an American psychologist who undertook a PhD in this field, lists five characteristics of clinical intuition as being 'sudden recognition, immediate knowledge, emergent awareness, non-verbal insight (such as in dreams) and holisitic, integrative sensibilities'.[24] She also highlights the importance of empathy, creativity, humour and compassion in the clinical intuitive process, and of adopting an open and curious frame of mind, being grounded in inner sensory faculties, and receiving information consciously to prepare the mind for deeper connections to the client. This is described as a 'being with' rather than 'doing to' mode of interaction.[25]

Marks-Tarlow suggests six ways to set the foundation for intuitive awareness:

1. Practise focus (through yoga, meditation, quiet sitting).
2. Open up your receptivity to inner emotional, sensory and body-based cues.
3. Develop a ritual for grounding and consulting your intuition, such as meditation.
4. Contact your inner signals; for example, pay attention to your body during a session with a client, without analyzing what is happening.
5. Clarify your values as a clinician.
6. Set intentions for yourself, for example, healing, empathizing and being authentic.[26]

You might want to explore this topic further. For my book, *Intuition: Unlock the power!* I researched the area of intuition and looked at its applications in the area of healing. The book identifies a number of steps to develop your intuition further:

- Make space for intuition in our lives, for example, through de-cluttering our schedules and our minds.
- Connect with yourself and others through being aware of values, connecting with your body, mind and spirit, and utilizing empathy.
- Practise meditation and mindfulness; inner stillness is important to connecting with your intuition.
- Enhance your creativity; creativity and intuition enhance each other.
- Access your unconscious mind through meditation, as well as understanding signs and symbols and our dreams. (an T)
- Tap into positivity; we know that positive emotions open us up to intuition, and we can cultivate these through kindness, gratitude and positive thinking.
- Apply intuition in your everyday and working life.

When working with clients on self-awareness, I often tap into these steps, and utilize the helpful exercises in the middle section of *Intuition*.

Reflection on Rosie's story

As Rosie continued her placement, the supervisor helped her become aware of her existing strengths and skills, and to develop more skills in relating to her client, such as listening carefully, establishing a therapeutic relationship and tapping into her intuition.

As a result Rosie's confidence grew, and this enabled her to further develop her counselling skills.

The integrative approach

The LLCC framework takes an integrative approach, combining different orientations or therapies.[27] I have adopted this approach for most of my working life, and view it as utilizing a range of philosophies, approaches and therapies to assist the whole person to manage their concerns and to bring about meaningful change in their life. This approach stems from my background as an OT and later as a GP, being careful to consider each aspect of the individual, whether physical, emotional, psycho-social, cultural, spiritual or vocational. Over the years I have been drawn to a number of therapies and I have also explored various philosophies, from Buddhism to existentialism, which have influenced my therapeutic approach. The concept that each individual is unique and therefore that one approach will not suit everyone works against adopting just one approach; plus, various types of therapy have both strengths and weaknesses.

The LLCC approach involves utilizing a range of therapies and philosophies to assist the whole person to manage their concerns and bring about meaningful change.

The integrative approach allows counsellors to look across a range of different schools of thought, and to be open to different perspectives. There is also what is known as **technical integration**, which involves selecting the best treatment techniques for the individual or the problem.[28] An example of this is Multimodal Therapy (MMT), developed by Arnold Lazarus, who recognized that individuals are unique and have different biological make-ups and personalities.[29] In its pure form, MMT adopts techniques from a range of therapies including Gestalt, Cognitive Behavioural, Psychodynamic and Family Systems Therapy. The decision as to which techniques to use is based on research as to what works best with the problems the client presents with, and on what seems best for the individual client. In other words, the therapist asks themself, 'What is best for this particular person?'[30]

A number of counselling texts, such as those written by psychologist and university professor Gerald Corey, are founded on an integrated approach. In fact, Corey suggests we remain open and 'selectively incorporate a framework for counselling that is consistent with [our] own personality and [our] belief system'.[31] In addition, it is interesting to note that some of the newer therapies such as Acceptance and Commitment Therapy (ACT) are in fact integrative therapies, borrowing from a range of therapies and philosophies. As we continue to consider assessment and management approaches, you will begin to understand that an integrated approach can be applied to counselling, and you will begin to identify what suits your practice and style. This is the very essence of the LLCC approach.

Consumer and carer perspectives

It is important to be mindful of appreciating what is important to clients or consumers, and their carers, and be aware of their perspectives and views, as they are the directors of their own care. Over the years of working with consumers and carers, both clinically and in teaching, a number of key issues have been highlighted. Reflect on these as you read them.

Key points from mental health clients include the following:

- Clients might not have a regular GP or counsellor, and they might find it hard to link in with one. They may need assistance to locate appropriate assistance.
- It is important to acknowledge the amount of effort it may have taken for the person to simply get to their appointment with you.
- Good communication skills (rapport, trust, listening, empathy, reassurance, repetition) are central. Listen to what the person is saying; value and acknowledge them.
- Recognize the client might be anxious about seeing a counsellor.
- It is important to provide time to talk and get to know the person.
- Be a partner in care. That is, talk with the person (not at or over them) and involve them in decision-making processes.
- Some clients report that they have been treated with less respect and dignity than they would want. Always treat the client as you would want to be treated.
- Obtain consent to collect information from other sources if appropriate (such as hospital, psychiatrist, mental health service, family member).
- Encourage self-management and self-empowerment (for example, 'It must be distressing to be where you are right now, but I have confidence that you will work out what you need').
- Provide information and support.
- Don't forget about the client's physical health needs.
- Liaise with other health professionals/carers involved in the person's care.
- Be aware of potential barriers to accessing assistance and services.
- Referral to non-government (NGO) and consumer organizations can be valuable.
- It is vital to maintain a sense of hope, and to carry out follow-up.

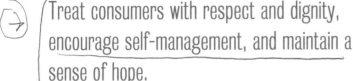

Treat consumers with respect and dignity, encourage self-management, and maintain a sense of hope.

Key points from mental health carers include the following:

- Good communication skills (rapport, trust, listening, empathy, reassurance, repetition) are central. Listen to what the person is saying; value and acknowledge their role.
- Assist carers in learning new communication skills to make communicating with the person they care for more effective.
- It is important to provide time to talk and get to know the person.
- Be a partner in care. That is, involve carers whenever possible.
- Carers often feel 'in the dark' and appreciate the provision of information and support wherever possible.
- Treat the carer with respect; validating their role is very important.
- Encourage self-empowerment and self-care, including managing stress and maintaining hobbies that are sustaining.
- Provide information and support.
- Be aware of potential barriers to accessing assistance and services.
- Referral to NGOs and carer organisations can be valuable.

> Carers appreciate the provision of information and support wherever possible.

Cultural and gender issues

It is essential to be aware of the influences of culture and gender in your society, and where you stand in relation to these. Many of us live in a multicultural society and racism exists. Counsellors will have their own unique life experiences that will have an impact on their attitudes, and it is important to examine and monitor these. We may fall into traps such as judging or stereotyping. The aim is not for the counsellor to feel guilty, but to be more consciously aware.[32] If relevant, it can be helpful to talk about cultural differences at the outset with a client, and to learn more about what has influenced them. This will lead to a more effective relationship between counsellor and client.[33] Many concepts such as self-disclosure and seeking help are culturally bound, and you might need to be open and flexible in your own approach. **Cultural empathy** refers to appreciating the world of the client, and understanding the attitudes expressed instead of simply observing them. It is also about offering this understanding to the client, with the willingness to be corrected. Palmer cites Ridley's tips for counselling clients from diverse cultural backgrounds:

- Develop cultural self-awareness.
- Avoid value imposition.

- Accept your naivety as a multicultural counsellor.
- Show cultural empathy.
- Incorporate cultural considerations into counselling.
- Do not stereotype.
- Determine the relative importance of the client's primary cultural roles.
- Do not blame the victim.
- Remain flexible in your selection of interventions.
- Examine your counselling theories for bias.
- Build on your client's strengths.
- Do not protect clients from emotional pain.[34]

In the area of mental health it is important to understand how individuals from other cultures perceive mental illness. There may also be particular healing practices within cultures.[35] Understanding the following principles can assist you in this area:

- Individualism versus collectivism. Western countries such as Australia and the United Kingdom are individualist countries, with personal achievement, personal choices and freedoms emphasized above group goals. Most Asian cultures are collectivist, that is, family and community goals are emphasized above individual needs or wants.
- Materialism versus spiritualism, where materialism refers to belief in the existence of the material world, and belief in non-material things is viewed as unscientific or superstitious. This is the dominant view in the West. Spiritualism is the dominant view in countries such as India, and may influence views about mental illness, for example.
- Cognitivism versus emotionalism. Cognitivism emphasizes the rational and logical, work and achievement, and emotions are to be kept in check. Emotionalism emphasizes feelings and intuition, and relationships.

Counsellors must also examine their views on gender and sexuality. Different societies will promote different views, and we are all influenced by these during our lives. Western cultures, for example, view the strengths of men and women as being different, influencing socialization practices and the roles we adopt during our lives. Consider society's views of the 'ideal' young woman (pretty, slim, competent, caring . . .) or young man (strong, muscular, breadwinner, successful . . .) and how these arise. Society also has had varying views on hetero and homosexuality. Not that long ago homosexuality was illegal in western countries, and was 'treated' with hormones and shock treatment, whereas now the legalization of marriage between same-sex couples is on the rise.

Women's movements in the late 1800s and the 1960s challenged the traditional ways of viewing women and their roles and power in society. In the early years of psychiatry, male gender-role traits were viewed as 'normative' whereas women's behaviours were more prone to be pathologized.[36] I certainly remember being taught various theories about the role of mothers in the causation of various mental illnesses during my early training. Therapy based on feminism, however, is about empowerment of women, and developing greater joy, self-confidence and self-acceptance.[37]

In discussion of feminist theory, Corey outlines the following useful principles.

- The personal is political.
- There is a commitment to social change.
- Female voices are valued, and their experiences honoured.
- The counselling relationship is egalitarian.
- Focus on strength. Reformulated definition of psychological distress.
- All types of oppression are recognized.[38]

Understanding socio-political influences underpins Narrative Therapy. It can be helpful in counselling to identify and validate the messages the client has received in terms of gender and sexuality, and the various expectations placed upon them. It is vital to be aware of feminist theory and gender in couple work. Counsellors can advocate for and assist the client to feel empowered, and assist them to define themselves rather than being defined by society. They can also teach the client skills such as assertiveness, which can assist in redressing power imbalances. Group work around these issues can also be particularly useful to draw upon shared experiences and to practise skills.

In summary

Caring is at the core of effective counselling, along with establishing a trusting relationship with clients and communicating effectively with them. It is through the therapeutic relationship that the client feels safe to express themselves, and together the counsellor and client can identify and use the client's own expertise and resources, and thereby foster their ability to change and grow.

The LLCC framework involves an integrative approach, adopting a range of philosophies, approaches and therapies to assist the whole person to manage their concerns. Central to the LLCC approach are the roles of caring and the therapeutic relationship, and unique is the inclusion of making use of your clinical intuition skills, which can provide valuable information.

Being respectful and involving clients and carers is vital in the counselling process, as is self-reflection. It is through self-reflection that the counsellor can grow in awareness of their own attitudes, such as to gender, sexuality and culture, which may influence their relationships and work with clients.

Resources

Corey, G. 2013, *Theory and Practice of Counseling and Psychotherapy (9th ed.),* Cengage Learning, California.

Howell, C. 2013, *Intuition: Unlock the power!* Exisle Publishing, New South Wales.

Hutchinson, D. 2015, *The Essential Counsellor Process, Skills and Techniques* (3rd ed.), Sage Publishing, Los Angeles.

Marks-Tarlow, T. 2012, *Clinical Intuition in Psychotherapy: The neurobiology of embodied response*, W.W. Norton & Company, New York.

Palmer, S. (ed.) 2002, *Multicultural Counselling*, Sage Publishing, London.

Chapter 2
The initial phase of counselling

A journey of a thousand leagues begins beneath one's feet.

—LAO TZU

The initial phase involves developing the therapeutic relationship. Historically, it did not necessarily incorporate a formal assessment process. However, an assessment is highly valuable and an essential part of practice. This chapter outlines the **LLCC assessment and management planning process,** which involves a comprehensive approach to gathering information, and developing a 'formulation' or understanding about the individual and their reasons for presenting. Management planning follows on from the assessment, and this incorporates values-based goal-setting. The LLCC assessment and management plan can be adapted to suit your practice, and can take a number of sessions to complete. The counsellor can pace this process to suit the client and their own style.

As you read the following case study, reflect on how a thorough assessment and management planning would assist the client, Sophie. The sections on genograms, formulation and management planning will refer back to her story.

(Note that in a later chapter on stress and anxiety, strategies for managing panic episodes will be outlined.)

Sophie's story

Sophie, 25 years old, presents feeling stressed and worried, particularly about several recent panic attacks. She has struggled with anxiety since her teens but started having panic episodes 6 months ago. Sophie lives with her partner, Brett, who is supportive. She studied business at university and now has her own business and also helps Brett with his. She grew up in the country and went to boarding school for the final years of her schooling. She found this stressful and did not feel like she fitted in at the school. Sophie has struggled with self-confidence since this time, despite achieving highly.

Sophie describes a strong relationship with her mother, but a sometimes difficult relationship with her father. He has periods of depression and Sophie hates it when he is critical of her. There was an argument a month ago and Sophie and her father are now not talking, and Sophie is having more frequent panic episodes. An assessment tool gives scores consistent with severe stress and anxiety.

The LLCC assessment

The assessment is a multifaceted process. It involves getting to know the client and building the therapeutic relationship, while understanding both the issues they are grappling with and their background. It involves taking the whole person into account and how they are functioning in each area of their life. When you meet with a client, you listen to their stories, the context they live in, their viewpoints and their intentions. The assessment might involve talking with family members or carers, or other counsellors or health professionals, if relevant and with the client's permission. The assessment phase also includes beginning to make plans about working together.

When you meet with a client, you listen to their stories, the context they live in, their viewpoints and their intentions.

Different authors have written about the stages in the counselling process. Egan speaks of the stages being as follows:

1. Clarification of the key issues calling for change by helping clients tell their story, develop new perspectives and focus on issues that will make a difference.

2. Helping clients determine preferred outcomes by considering what they want, then translating these into goals, and consideration of what they are willing to pay for what they want, in terms of effort and commitment to goals.

3. Helping clients develop and plan strategies to accomplishing their goals.[1]

At the outset it is essential for counsellors to discuss **confidentiality** with clients. For adult clients, confidentiality can be explained by saying: 'It is important for you [the client] to be aware that what is discussed in the sessions is confidential to yourself and myself [the counsellor], unless there is concern about risk of harm to yourself or others. Then I [the counsellor] have a duty of care to act on this information which may involve informing others.' For young people, parental consent is needed for treatment at certain ages, and I recommend you refer to the relevant legislation for your state or country

of residence. For a client of any age it can be useful to add that if there is anything they do not feel comfortable talking about, they can ask you to leave the subject. You will need to use your judgment as to the need to come back to the topic later, or whether it can be left entirely.

At the outset it is essential for counsellors to discuss confidentiality with clients.

The assessment of the client, their needs and situation, needs to be thorough and comprehensive. You will need to adapt the LLCC assessment to your area of practice. The importance of a good assessment cannot be overemphasized, and the following steps can assist with this:

1. Have a new client form to collect their general details (personal details including date or birth, contact details and next of kin) and referral details.

2. Discuss and record the client's main concerns in detail, including the timeframe and current stressors.

3. Enquire about relevant history, such as previous experience of similar issues, past experience of counselling, relevant past medical history (such as recent or chronic illness, or recent childbirth), and mental health history (such as past depression or anxiety).

4. If relevant to your field, find out if the client is taking regular medication (prescribed or over the counter, such as supplements) and ask about substance use (e.g. tobacco, alcohol, illicit drugs).
5. Explore the client's personal and social history, beginning with drawing a **genogram** or visual representation of an individual's biological and legal family from generation to generation, and finding out about the family structure.

THE GENOGRAM

Genograms give a graphical depiction of individuals in a person's family, and the lines between these indicate the relationship experienced with them. Genograms can guide the counsellor in relation to the strength and quality of relationships that the individual has had with significant others throughout their lives, and how past generations might influence the present.[2] There are recognized symbols to use in creating genograms, as shown in Figure 1.

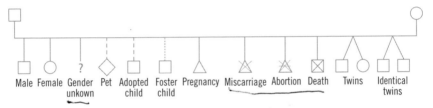

Figure 1: Genogram symbols[3]

For couples and relationships there are standard symbols: a dotted line between individuals represents distance between the two, a jagged line represents a hostile relationship, and so on.

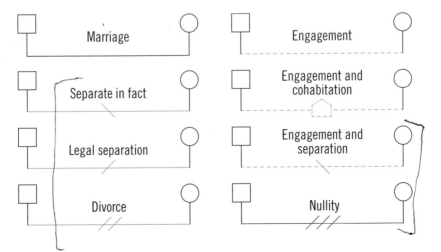

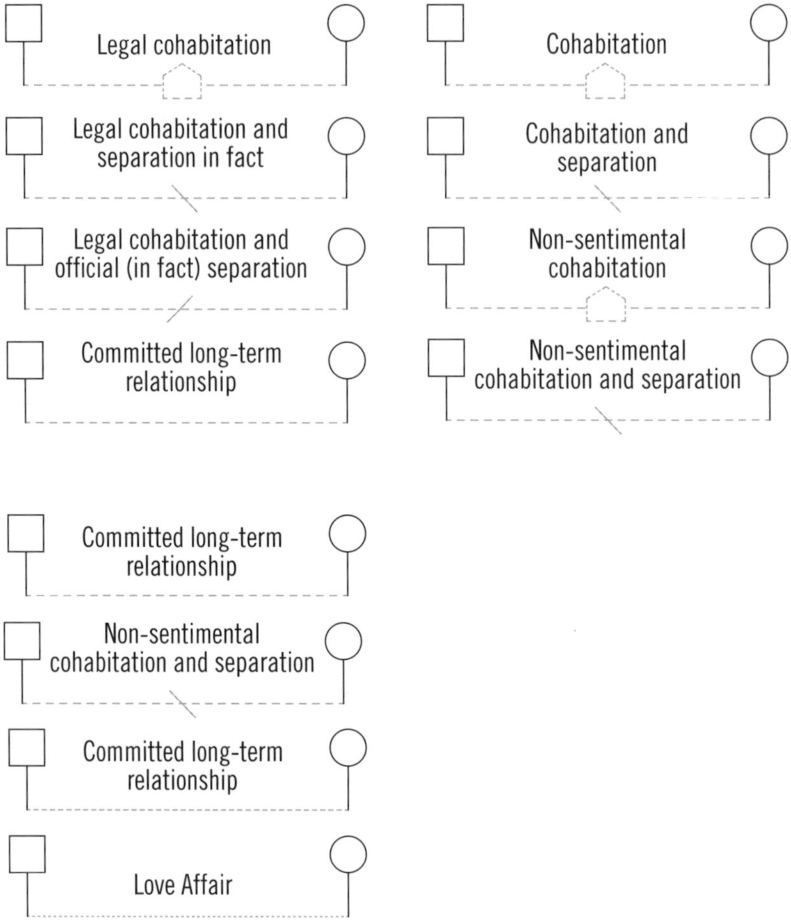

Figure 2: Representing relationships on the genogram

Here is a sample genogram, based on Sophie's story.

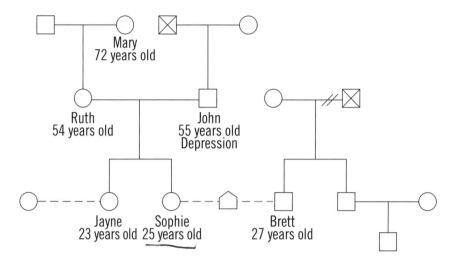

Figure 3: Sophie's genogram

Once you have completed the client's genogram, move on to the following points.

- Enquire about:
    - the client's place of birth (they may have immigrated) and culture
    - their childhood, including their experience with primary school, their friendships and interests
    - their experience of high school and adolescence (note any issues becoming apparent in adolescence such as gender identity issues)
    - any important family events, and history of grief or trauma
    - aspects of adulthood, such as work or education, living arrangements, interests and leisure activities
    - further relationship history with family, work colleagues, friends and partner relationships (present, past, same sex).
- Establish any **risk factors** (such as family history of mental health issues, recent stresses or traumas) and protective factors (including past coping skills, positive social support, employment or financial stability).
- Consider strategies or therapies that have previously been helpful to the client.
- Enquire about any other areas you believe are relevant to that individual.

MENTAL STATE EXAMINATION

When assessing an individual presenting with a mental health issue, it will be relevant for some health professionals or counsellors to undertake a **Mental State Examination** (MSE) as part of the assessment. This involves assessing the client in relation to:

- appearance, for example, neatly dressed or dishevelled
- behaviour, such as agitated or distracted
- conversation, whether appropriate, flowing or otherwise
- affect, such as depressed, reactive, quite expressionless or flat
- perception, that is, presence or absence of hallucinations or delusions
- cognition, which includes memory, orientation, attention, thinking
- insight, judgment, intelligence and rapport.

All counsellors must have skills in **risk assessment** (for factors such as self-harm and suicide). This will be addressed in Part 3.

Take some time now to consider what questions you might use during this assessment. Here are some ideas.

- 'How are you feeling at the moment? Can you rate that feeling on a scale of 0 to 10 [where 0 refers to having none of the feeling and 10 refers to the worst it could be]?'
- 'How long have you been feeling like this? When did you last feel okay?'
- 'How is your health generally? Have you had any recent illnesses? Are you taking any prescribed medications, or anything regularly from the pharmacy [including supplements]?'
- 'Do you smoke cigarettes, and [if yes] how many? Do you drink alcohol, and [if yes] how much would you drink over a week? Do you use any other drugs, such as marijuana or pills?'
- 'Let's start at the beginning. Where were you born? Who was in your family? Tell me about your parents, your siblings and grandparents. Was there anyone else who was significant growing up?'
- 'What sort of person was your mother/father? How did everyone get on at home?'
- 'How was your childhood — was it fairly happy or unhappy? Describe your life at home.'

- 'Can you tell me about school? What about friendships? What were you interested in growing up? Did you experience any bullying?'
- 'Were there any memorable events growing up? Did you experience any grief or traumatic events? If you had to relive your childhood, would you want anything changed?'
- 'Tell me about your adolescence. How was school at this time, and friendships? Were there any struggles in relation to sexuality or gender?'
- 'Do you have a partner? Can you tell me about them? Can you tell me about previous partner relationships?'
- 'Are you working? If so, what sort of work do you do? Do you have any financial worries?'
- 'Is there anything else on your mind at moment? Are there any other stresses currently?'
- 'Have we missed anything else that you think is important to mention? [or] Is there anything else you haven't been able to tell me as yet? You don't have to necessarily tell me now, but we could flag the issue to come back to later if you like.'

Assessment tools

You may choose to utilize **assessment tools** to add to your understanding of the client's story and issues. It is important to remember that assessment tools assist, but do not replace, your professional judgment.

Assessment tools can be used for screening, as an aid to diagnosis, or for monitoring severity of the problem. (Full versions of the K10, DASS and HEADSS assessment tools mentioned below can be found in the Appendix, beginning on p. 281, along with a pro forma for the LLCC assessment and management plan.)

SCREENING

Screening tools are designed to see if the condition is likely in a population. An example is the FEAR questionnaire screening for anxiety, where F stands for frequency of worry ('How often, if at all, have you been worried in the past month?'); E for the enduring nature of anxiety ('In general, have you always been a worrier?'); A for alcohol/sedative use to reduce anxiety ('Do you use alcohol or other substances to help you cope with your worry?'); and R stands for restlessness or fidgeting ('In the past month, have you felt so fidgety or restless that you could not sit still?'). The scoring for this tool is straightforward: a positive response to one or more of the four questions indicates a 74 per cent chance of having an anxiety disorder.[4]

The Kessler or K10 is another example of a screening tool. It measures levels of psychological distress based on ten questions about anxiety and depressive symptoms that a person has experienced in the last four weeks. Each item is scored from 1, which is used to indicate 'none of the time', to 5, which is used to indicate 'all of the time'. Scores of the ten items are added together, giving a minimum score of 10 and a maximum of 50. Low scores indicate low levels of psychological distress, and high scores indicate high levels of psychological distress. As a guide, when the score is 17 or above on the K10, further clinical assessment should be undertaken to identify the nature of the psychological distress the person is experiencing and to assess the risk of self-harm and suicide.[5] It is also worth looking at the Primary Care Evaluation of Mental Disorders (Prime-MD), another validated screening tool available in the public domain.[6]

DIAGNOSIS

Diagnostic tools have been devised and validated in different communities to enable their use in diagnosing particular mental health problems, such as depression. One example is the Depression, Anxiety and Stress Scale (DASS), devised by Australian academic psychologist Peter Lovibond. The DASS assesses an individual's rate of depression, anxiety and stress, categorizing their scores into normal, mild, moderate, severe and extremely severe levels. It comes in 21-item and 42-item self-report versions, and asks patients to reflect on the past week. The DASS has the benefit of providing a measure of depression, anxiety and stress in a single test.[7]

MONITORING

The DASS is an example of a measuring tool that can also be used to monitor severity of symptoms, and is very useful to use regularly over time, to help monitor the client's progress.

The K10 can also be used for monitoring progress, and there a range of other tools such as the Hamilton Depression Rating Scale, the Beck Anxiety Scale and the Geriatric Depression Scale.

Some assessment tools require further training or qualifications in order to be used. And be aware, too, that the client's age and cultural background will influence which tool you might utilize. For example, for young people, a HEADSS assessment is useful, where:

H = home
E = education, employment, eating and exercise
A = activities, hobbies and peer relationships
D = drug use

S = sexual activity and sexuality

S = suicide, depression and mental health, safety/risk.[8]

Formulation

Once all of the history has been completed, the next step is to pull together the information into a **formulation** about 'aetiology' or causation, to help you and the client understand their presentation and the reasons for the issues they are presenting with. The aetiology formulation addresses the question: 'Why is this patient suffering from this/these problem/s at this point in time?' It allows you to integrate the information that has been gathered, linking its different aspects to come to an understanding of the unique individual, with their vulnerabilities and resources. Later you can also create a management formulation or plan.

There are various models for formulations, and some therapies have their own, such as MMT, Cognitive Behaviour Therapy (CBT), ACT and Interpersonal Therapy (IPT). It is worth exploring all of these, but in LLCC the focus will be on two general and useful formulation models, the first of which incorporates 'the five Ps', namely: presenting issues, precipitating, predisposing, perpetuating and protective factors for the issues.

- **Presenting issues** are those concerns described by the client when they initially come to you.
- **Predisposing factors** are those factors in the client's history that make them susceptible or inclined towards the current distress or mental health problem.
- **Precipitating factors** are the immediate factors that have caused the client to come to you. Note, however, that two different people would likely react differently to the same factors or circumstances, depending on background, life experience, supports, coping strategies and current circumstances.
- **Perpetuating factors** are those that are causing the client's symptoms to continue or worsen.
- **Protective factors** include the factors that protect the client and enhance resilience, such as good social support or employment.[9]

The second model is known as **BPSSC** and defines the **b**iological, **p**sychological, **s**ocial, **s**piritual and **c**ultural forces that have contributed towards the development of the client's concerns and their response to them. It is holistic in nature. Here are some examples of how the BPSSC factors might influence the individual and their distress.

1. Biological:
   - genetic factors (family history of illness)

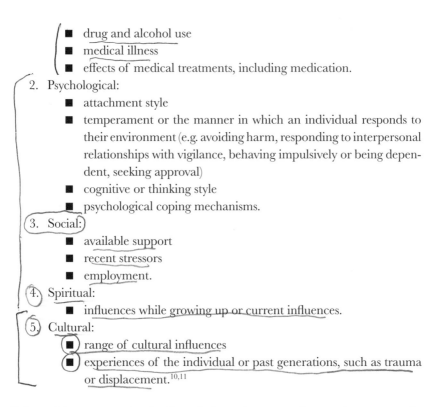

- drug and alcohol use
- medical illness
- effects of medical treatments, including medication.

2. Psychological:
   - attachment style
   - temperament or the manner in which an individual responds to their environment (e.g. avoiding harm, responding to interpersonal relationships with vigilance, behaving impulsively or being dependent, seeking approval)
   - cognitive or thinking style
   - psychological coping mechanisms.

3. Social:
   - available support
   - recent stressors
   - employment.

4. Spiritual:
   - influences while growing up or current influences.

5. Cultural:
   - range of cultural influences
   - experiences of the individual or past generations, such as trauma or displacement.[10,11]

It is useful to summarize the formulation using a template such as the one in Figure 4. This is based on the BPSSC model and the formulation used in IPT, and it allows you to incorporate the five Ps. It will assist you to pull together the information with the client, and the visual representation often aids the client's understanding and is reassuring for them: 'It makes sense now that I can see it in this way' is a typical comment.

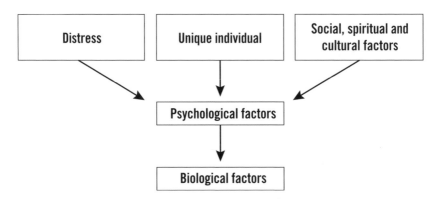

Figure 4: A formulation template[12]

Now recall Sophie's story. The formulation for Sophie might look like this:

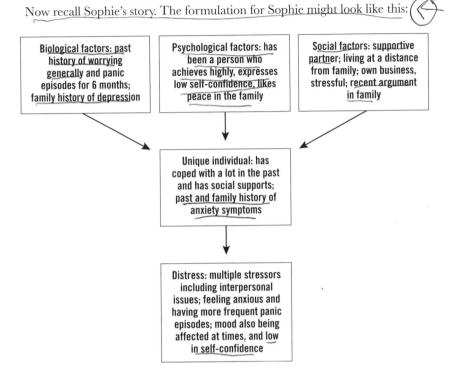

Figure 5: Sophie's formulation

Management planning

Once the assessment has been completed, the next step is to work collaboratively with the client to develop a **management plan**. Planning involves identifying:

- the key issues or problems
- goals
- approaches, therapies or strategies to be used.

It also includes having a crisis plan and a relapse prevention plan.

The management plan is not fixed in stone, and you will no doubt deviate from the plan to explore ideas, problems or issues that might arise. However, it provides a guide for the counsellor and client about what will be worked on together, and it allows discussion about what the client sees as their main need/s or key issues. It also enables you to explore what they see as priorities to address early on, and what you view as most important. This can be discussed and together you can prioritize the issues.

A table for management planning is included in the LLCC assessment and management plan pro forma in the Appendix (see p. 293). Here is an example of a completed plan for Sophie.

Table 1: Sophie's management plan

Client needs/issues/ problems (prioritized)	Goals	Approaches/ therapies/ strategies
• Anxiety — worrying generally and having panic episodes • Interpersonal distress (recent conflict) • Significant stress (business, living at distance from family . . .) • Mood being impacted — increasingly low mood • Low self-confidence	• Learn strategies to reduce worrying • Learn strategies to deal with panic episodes • Work through the interpersonal issues • Explore causes of stress • Reduce stress level • Monitor and improve mood • Improve self-confidence and self-belief	• Support • Psycho-education • Counselling • Interpersonal strategies (managing conflict) • CBT, ACT, Narrative Therapy, Hypnotherapy • Highlight strengths, ways to tap into positivity • Strategies to improve self-belief and self-confidence

During this phase you may want to spend more time in the planning process to really identify and focus on what is important in life to the client; in other words, their **values**. This brings more meaning to the planning and transforms it into more of a therapeutic process. In addition, the following ideas based on ACT provide the client with a clear idea about the steps they are going to take in order to manage the issues.[13] To begin this process, ask the client to consider what they value in life, or what is important to them, and explain that this might relate to what they want their life to be about, what sort of person they want to be or what relationships they want to build. Introduce the different areas or domains in life, namely:

- family and friends
- romance or intimate relationships
- health and the body
- education and personal development
- work and finance
- leisure

- citizenship or community life
- environment or nature
- spirituality.[14,15]

Then ask the client to consider their values in relation to each of these domains. Table 2 can assist; it provides the domain headings, and under each heading the client can list what is valued or important to them. The left-hand column is completed first. For example, under the heading of work, having a job and job satisfaction might be important.

The next step is to complete the column on the right, asking whether there is gap between what is important and what is actually happening currently. There will be some domains in which the client feels their current life is pretty consistent with what they value. For example, they might value spending time with family and friends and that might be what is happening. However, in other areas, there might be a gap between what is important to them and what is currently happening; for example, they might value fitness but currently do not spend much time doing exercise. The gaps can then be highlighted in the table. A copy is provided in the Appendix (see p. 295).

Table 2: Life domains and values

Domain	'What is important to you/what do you value in this domain?'	'Is there a gap between what is currently happening and what you value?'
Family and friends		
Romance/intimate relationships		
Health and your body		
Education and personal development		
Work and finance		
Leisure (for example, hobbies, relaxation time)		

Citizenship/community life (such as helping a neighbour, volunteering)		
Environment or nature		
Spirituality		

GOALS

Having completed the table, consider those domains in which gaps are present. Ask the client to consider which of these is particularly important to them at this time, and which domains they want to focus on at the moment. These ideas will help the client and the counsellor identify goals. It is useful to:

- make a goals list with the client
- encourage goals which are the client's own, as well as goals that are specific, potentially measurable, achievable, realistic and time-based
- prioritize the goals in terms of importance and available energy/resources
- break down the prioritized goal into small steps.

Table 3 gives an example of how a client might record their goal and how they will achieve it.[16]

Table 3: Goal-setting

My goal is:
To work towards my goal, my first step will be:
• Second step:
• Third step:
• Fourth step:
Benefits from achieving this goal:
The time, day, date for taking the first step:
I will know I have achieved my goal because:

As an example, let's take one of Sophie's goals and use this format.

Table 4: Sophie's goals

My goal is: *to learn strategies to reduce worrying*

To work towards my goal, my first step will be: *to practise several breathing techniques each day*

- Second step: *to keep a diary recording when and how often I practise*
- Third step: *practise, practise!*
- Fourth step: *I will also write down any worries before I go to sleep*

Benefits from achieving this goal: *I will worry less over time*

The time, day, date for taking the first step: *Today, Monday at 10 a.m.*

I will know I have achieved my goal because: *I am keeping a diary of the breathing practice, and writing down how I feel each day*

A CRISIS PLAN

Counsellors need to discuss with clients what might constitute a crisis, and what they would do to keep themselves supported and safe in such an event. Strategies might involve contacting family members, a supportive friend, various community help phone lines, mental health services or emergency services. The counsellor might make themselves available for contact at certain times, and this will vary depending on the setting the counsellor is working in. The crisis plan with contact details should be documented on the management plan.

RELAPSE PREVENTION PLANNING

Relapse prevention planning may be another vital aspect of the management plan. There are three steps in developing a plan for managing relapse, and depression and anxiety are used as an example here:

1. **Identify the early warning symptoms**, such as difficulty sleeping, ruminating, more panic attacks.
2. **Identify possible high-risk situations** for relapse, such as stress or being overtired. Consider strategies for the client to protect themself, for example, relaxation or mindfulness techniques.
3. **Prepare an emergency plan** to put into action when the depression is relapsing, such as monitoring thinking, getting support from friends

or family, making an earlier (or urgent) appointment with the GP or counsellor.[17]

In summary

The initial phase of counselling involves assessment and management planning. The LLCC assessment provides a comprehensive assessment, an essential part of the counselling process. Information is gathered by the counsellor through hearing the client's story and asking questions about their background and the current issues, and includes a risk assessment. Assessment tools can be used to provide further information. The aim is to develop a formulation or understanding about the individual and their reasons for presenting.

Management planning follows on from the assessment, and this provides a guide for the counsellor and client about what will be worked on together. It enables discussion about what the client sees as the key issues and incorporates values-based goal-setting. Once the assessment and plan is complete, the counsellor and client are then able to move forward into working through the key issues.

Reflection on Sophie's story

The counsellor spent several sessions hearing Sophie's story and carefully working through the LLCC assessment. Sophie appreciated the opportunity to share her concerns, and to understand the various factors contributing to her distress. The management plan clarified the key issues and Sophie was keen to begin work on the first goal of learning strategies to reduce worrying.

Early on, the counsellor taught Sophie breathing and relaxation techniques and over further sessions they continued to work through the issues with a range of approaches and therapies. Central to recovery was addressing the distressing interpersonal issue.

Resources

Books

Corey, G. 2013, *Theory and Practice of Counseling and Psychotherapy (9th ed.)*, Cengage Learning, California.

Egan, G. 2007, *The Skilled Helper: A problem-management and opportunity development approach to helping (8th ed.)*, Brooks/Cole Publishing, USA.

Harris, R. 2009, *ACT Made Simple: An easy-to-read primer on Acceptance and Commitment Therapy*, New Harbinger Publications, California.

Howell, C. 2010, *Keeping the Blues Away: A guide to preventing relapse of depression*, Radcliffe, London.

Howell, C. and Murphy, M., 2011, *Release Your Worries: A guide to letting go of stress and anxiety*, Exisle Publishing, New South Wales.

McGoldrick, M. and Gerson, R. 2008, *Genograms in Family Assessment*, W.W. Norton & Company, New York.

Weissman M., Markowitz, J. and Klerman G. 2007, *Clinician's Quick Guide to Interpersonal Psychotherapy*, Oxford University Press.

Websites

ACT: www.actmindfully.com.au

DASS: http://www2.psy.unsw.edu.au/dass/

Formulation: www.psychtraining.org/RANZCP-Formulations-Guide.pdf

Genograms: www.genograms.org/symbols/

IPT: www.interpersonalpsychotherapy.org

Relapse prevention: www.drcatehowell.com.au

Chapter 3
The LLCC integrative approach

Happiness is not a state to arrive at, rather,
a manner of travelling.
—SAMUEL JOHNSON

The LLCC approach draws on a range of philosophies, approaches and therapies. As highlighted earlier, this is an integrative approach, which allows counsellors to be open to different philosophies and perspectives, and to adopt a range of therapeutic approaches. One philosophy already highlighted is caring for the whole person by considering biological, psychological, social, spiritual and cultural aspects of the person. This chapter outlines the other philosophies, approaches and therapies which have influenced the LLCC approach, and also explores a number of therapies which have been incorporated into the LLCC approach. It is these which will be applied in Part 2, which is all about managing key life issues and problem areas.

Read the following story. John's situation is complex, and there are many factors to consider. As you read this chapter, consider how some of the philosophies, approaches or therapies might be relevant in working with John. His story will be reflected upon at the end of the chapter.

John's story

John grew up with his mother. His father was violent towards his mother and left the home when he was four years old. John is close to his mother but has had very little to do with his father since this time. He is married to Robyn and they have a two-year-old daughter, and another baby on the way. He loves spending time with his daughter, and is pleased she will have a sibling soon.

John works in sales, but his main interest in life is working with wood. He never had the chance to do a trade and would love to learn woodwork and wood-turning at some stage.

John has struggled with his mood since having children. He has felt the absence of his own father in his life more strongly. His irritability is now taking a toll on his relationship with his wife, and he is struggling with motivation at work.

Influential philosophies and approaches

During my career, I have been fascinated by the philosophies and approaches I have come across in formal and informal teaching, at conferences, in supervision and in my reading. I will touch on some of those that have influenced the development of the LLCC approach.

PERSON-CENTRED THERAPY AND HUMANISTIC PSYCHOLOGY

Ideas from both these approaches have already been addressed, in particular, the unconditional positive regard for the client and the therapeutic relationship. Rogers developed person-centred therapy, which has a focus on the resources people have within themselves and the potential for growth. Humanistic psychology has influenced many subsequent approaches and therapies, including taking a 'strengths-based approach' in counselling, and you will also see its influence on Narrative Therapy and Positive Psychology (more on these later in the chapter).

The strengths-based approach recognizes the **resilience** of individuals and focuses on their strengths, interests, abilities and capacities, rather than any limitations.[1] It is based on the principle that every individual, family and community has strengths, and all individuals have the capacity to learn and grow. The client is at the centre of counselling, and self-determination and responsibility is a key part of this approach.[2]

EXISTENTIALISM

Another influence in LLCC is existentialism. The existential movement respected the individual, and grew out of a desire to help people engage with life challenges and see the possibilities of being human.[3] It viewed individuals as constantly recreating themselves, through:

- self-awareness
- freedom and responsibility
- creating identity and relationships with others
- the search for meaning, purpose, values and goals
- anxiety as a condition of living
- awareness of death.[4]

Victor Frankl (1905–1997), one of the founders of Existential Therapy, was Jewish and experienced Hitler's concentration camps first-hand. He developed his own existential philosophy and therapy called Logotherapy ('therapy through meaning'), at the centre of which was the human will to find meaning, and the view that life has meaning under all circumstances.[5] The importance of **meaning** has been incorporated into a number of modern therapies including ACT and Narrative Therapy. It is also recognized as a major factor in developing positive emotions and is addressed in Positive Psychology. It is an integral part of the LLCC approach.

Humans search for meaning in life, and believe it has meaning under all circumstances. Meaning is a major factor in developing positive emotions.

ATTACHMENT THEORY

Attachment theory was first introduced by John Bowlby, a British psychiatrist, in the late 1950s. Attachment refers to an enduring emotional bond characterized by a tendency to seek and maintain closeness to a specific person, especially during times of stress. Bowlby based his theory on the observation of normal infant development and direct observation of parent–child interactions. Developing a secure attachment with caregivers is necessary for the development of our abilities to regulate our own emotions. When caregivers are responsive to their infant's needs, it provides a *safe base* for the infant to explore their world. When care is inconsistent or unresponsive, then anxious attachments can develop and the infant copes with separation by getting angry, overly clingy or being detached.[6]

Attachment theory has influenced a number of therapies, including Interpersonal Therapy (IPT), which focuses on interpersonal relationships. Early attachments shape our expectations in later relationships, and so this theory is important to understand when working with couples and families, as well as individuals. It is also relevant to the therapeutic relationship, as the aim is for the counsellor to provide a secure base to the client. This means they are reliable and responsive, and can work with negative emotions, especially in relation to separation or loss.[7]

MULTIMODAL THERAPY

The technically integrated approach taken in Multimodal Therapy (MMT) has influenced LLCC. Multimodal Therapy works across a range of modalities, namely human behaviour, affect (emotions), sensations (such as sight and hearing), imagery (including mental images of oneself and dreams), cognition, interpersonal relationships, drugs and other biological factors. The theory in MMT is that these modalities form a hierarchy, with interpersonal relationships at the top and biological influences at the base, and each is influenced by the others.

MMT suggests that unless all of these modalities are assessed, endeavours to change in therapy will be less likely. They provide a framework for assessment and management planning, and foster an eclectic approach to therapy, with the development of a tailored management plan for each client. MMT views therapy as an educational process, to facilitate learning and develop adaptive modes of responding. It draws freely from other schools of thought and uses homework, lifestyle measures and Bibliotherapy (self-help with books).[8]

Multimodal Therapy entails a tailored management plan for each client, and views therapy as an educational process.

MINDFULNESS

A philosophy that has come to prominence in the western world in the past twenty years is mindfulness. It is, however, thousands of years old and stems from Buddhist and Hindu practices. It refers to paying purposeful and non-judgmental attention to the present moment. In other words, mindfulness refers to focusing on what you are doing and experiencing in the present moment as opposed to thinking about the past or future.[9] For example, if you are brushing your teeth you are fully aware of and involved in every facet of the act of brushing your teeth.

A variety of mindfulness techniques have been incorporated into psychotherapy, such as mindful breathing, mindfulness meditation or everyday mindfulness (such as being in the present moment when doing everyday activities like walking). In a mindful state, neurons or nerve cells in the brain are activated, and growth is stimulated.[10] This is why several of the newer psychological approaches, such as Mindfulness-based Cognitive Therapy (MBCT) and Acceptance and Commitment Therapy (ACT), incorporate mindfulness.

Mindfulness refers to paying purposeful and non-judgmental attention to the present moment. The mindful state stimulates brain growth.

Mindfulness reminds us that the only moment over which we have any control is the present one. Australian GP, Dr Russ Harris, reports that practising mindfulness helps us to:

- be fully present in the moment
- experience unpleasant thoughts and feelings safely
- become aware of what feelings we are avoiding
- be more connected to ourselves, others and the wider world
- become less judgmental and increase self-awareness
- be less disturbed by and less reactive to unpleasant experiences
- learn the distinction between ourselves and our thoughts
- have more direct contact with the world, instead of living through thoughts
- learn that thoughts and feelings come and go
- have more balance and less emotional turmoil
- experience more calm and peacefulness
- develop self-acceptance and self-compassion.[11]

Note that having self-compassion is just like having compassion for others. It refers to being kind and understanding towards oneself when faced with personal failings, instead of being self-critical and judging oneself harshly.[12]

POSITIVE PSYCHOLOGY

In recent years, as a reaction against the focus on psychological disorders and illness, psychologist and researcher Martin Seligman created a new direction in psychology called Positive Psychology. It focuses on human strengths and virtues, and psychological wellbeing, and it aims to help people flourish or achieve an optimal level of health and wellbeing.[13] Positive Psychology seeks to investigate what people do correctly in life; that is, many people adapt to life in highly creative ways that allow them to feel good about life.[14]

Positive Psychology considers:

- positive subjective states, such as happiness, joy, love or confidence
- positive individual traits, for example, courage, persistence, honesty, sensitivity, maturity or wisdom
- positive associations including healthy families, institutions or communities.

Positive Psychology is the psychology of **PERMA**:

- **p**ositive emotions, such as joy or love
- **e**ngagement in life and activities
- **r**elationships
- **m**eaning in life
- **a**ccomplishment.

There are many benefits to positive psychology. According to Fredrickson, Positive Psychology:[15]

- changes the contents, scope and boundaries of your mind
- widens the span of possibilities
- 'undoes' the physiological effects of negativity
- feels good and transforms the future
- obeys a 'tipping point' — this refers to the ratio of positive to negative thoughts, as we need three positive thoughts for each negative one in order to flourish
- brings out the best in humans; that is, it opens up the capacity to build many resources including physical (for example, better sleep), mental (such as increased mindfulness), psychological (including optimism and resilience) and social (for example, better connections to friends and family).[16]

MOTIVATIONAL INTERVIEWING

Motivational Interviewing (MI) is not a therapy in own right but an approach that can be helpful at the outset of working with a client, to underpin later work. MI is a directive, client-centred counselling style that has been shown to be effective in its aim to bring about behaviour change.[17] Sometimes we feel ambivalent about change or we may actually resist change. We might have a degree of comfort or discomfort about how things are, and there might be discomfort about changing too. Motivational Interviewing helps individuals to explore and resolve this ambivalence.

In MI the counsellor avoids acting as an 'expert'. They listen and understand, but recognize that the individual needs to determine their own direction and goals.[18] The counsellor aims to pick up any discrepancy between what the client values or aims to change and the current problem behaviour. For example, an individual might use smoking as a way of dealing with stress; however, they might be worried about the effect of smoking on their lungs. The counsellor would help them identify these views, perhaps by looking at a future with the behaviour still present and one with the behaviour absent. They would also help the individual feel more confident that they can change, help them plan change and help them feel more optimistic about the change.[19,20]

Motivational Interviewing can underpin various therapies. It aims to bring about behaviour change.

As a counsellor, skills involved in MI include:
- expressing empathy
- helping the client develop discrepancy; that is, highlighting ambivalence about the behaviour
- rolling with any resistance from the client; that is, take a step back, approach the issue from another angle and ask the client's point of view
- supporting self-efficacy by developing the client's belief in their own ability to make changes, and reinforcing any successes.

Motivational Interviewing involves a series of steps, as follows:
- After assessment, ask the client's permission to talk about the issues identified.
- Explore the client's recognition of the issue/s as a problem.
- Assess their **readiness to change**: are they not at the stage of contemplating change; are they contemplating or making changes already; or are they at risk of relapse?
- Explore ambivalence by looking at the pros and cons of change (and of staying the same).

- Does the client believe they are able to make changes? Have they made changes before? What has gotten in the way?
- Is the client ready, willing and able to change?
- What are the next steps? What does the client think are the next steps?
- If appropriate, provide education to the client about the issues. Check they are happy to hear this information, and ask them what they already know about the issue. Take care not to overwhelm the client with information.
- If appropriate to their stage of change, you might use collaborative problem-solving (see p. 94).
- If appropriate to their stage of change, establish goals for change.
- If the client is not ready to change, leave the door open for them to come back to the issue/s.
- If the client is in relapse, it is important to look at their successes and at what has prevented continued success, and to use goals and problem-solving to help them get back on track.

The BATHE technique

The Bathe technique is separate to Motivational Interviewing, though it is a useful approach to mention. As with MI, the BATHE technique can be useful in early meetings with clients to aid communication and foster rapport. It involves the following steps, and can be repeated if and when needed.

- **B**ackground information to elicit context: 'What's brought you in?'
- **A**ffect, with a focus on mood: 'How has that made you feel?' 'What's your mood been like?'
- **T**roubling, to help to prioritize issues: 'What's troubling you most about this?'
- **H**andling, which moves the focus to client strengths and resources: 'How have you been handling that?'
- **E**mpathy to legitimizse feelings and convey concern: 'It sounds like it would've been really difficult.'[21]

The LLCC approach

It is from these various philosophies and approaches that some of the widely used modern-day therapies have been developed. We will now move onto describing a range of therapies, aspects of which have been incorporated into the LLCC approach, namely:

- Solution-focused Therapy (SFT)
- Cognitive Behaviour Therapy (CBT)

- Mindfulness-based Cognitive Therapy (MBCT)
- Acceptance and Commitment Therapy (ACT)
- Interpersonal Therapy (IPT)
- Narrative Therapy
- Hypnotherapy
- expressive therapies
- Positive Therapy
- Bibliotherapy and e-mental health.

While some of these therapies adopt perspectives and ideas that differ, this does not mean they cannot be useful in an integrative approach. As mentioned at the outset, 'one size does not fit all' and you will find that some clients find a particular approach extremely helpful but do not relate to another. For example, one client might find CBT useful but another will not relate to challenging their thoughts and instead, perhaps, find MBCT and ACT more relevant to them. With an integrative approach, the counsellor can adapt to the client and expose them to a number of therapies. Together the client and counsellor can then identify what is most helpful to that individual.

In the process of formalizing the ideas presented in this book, a **model** illustrating the key elements of the LLCC approach emerged. As you read the book, the key elements will come through as themes in the discussion. Consider the model in Figure 6 first. You will see that the client is at the centre of the model, and it also highlights the centrality of caring and the therapeutic relationship. Various aspects of the individual and their psyche are included in the model, such as life experiences, personality and strengths, as well as the client's thoughts, feelings and behaviours.

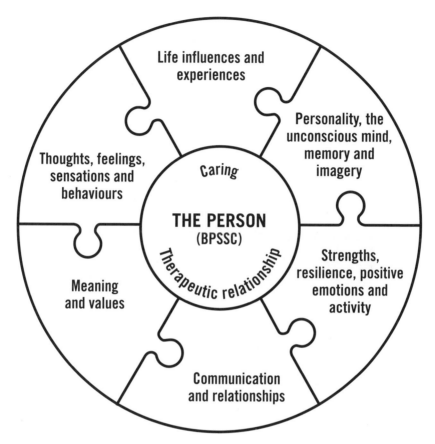

Figure 6: The LLCC model

Now consider Table 5 on the following page, which outlines the various philosophies, approaches and therapies, aspects of which have been integrated into the LLCC approach. For example, various therapies address the element of 'thoughts, feelings, sensations and behaviours', namely MI, CBT, MBCT, ACT, Bibliotherapy and e-mental health. There is some overlap as would be expected (for example, Narrative Therapy can be found under several of the key elements).

Table 5: The LLCC approach

LLCC key elements	Integrated philosophies, approaches and therapies
Meaning and values	Existentialism, Narrative Therapy, ACT, Positive Psychology
Life influences and experiences	Attachment theory, Narrative Therapy, CBT
Personality, the unconscious mind, memory and imagery	Clinical intuition, Hypnotherapy, ACT
Thoughts, feelings, sensations and behaviours	MI, CBT, MBCT, ACT, Hypnotherapy, expressive therapies, Bibliotherapy, e-mental health
Communication and relationships	IPT, couple therapy, Positive Psychology
Strengths, coping, resilience, positive emotions, activity	SFT, Narrative Therapy, Positive Psychology

The next section will provide background information on each of the therapies integrated into the LLCC approach. And in Part 2, the various therapies are applied in dealing with the various life issues and problem areas.

SOLUTION-FOCUSED THERAPY (SFT)

This is a brief collaborative approach focused on solutions, rather than the problem. It assumes the client wants to change, has the capacity to envisage change, is trying their best to make change happen and that the solution is already underway. It can be helpful when there is a pressing issue that needs to be addressed. Solution-focused Therapy considers what the client will do about the issues and how they will carry out their plans. It draws on the client's resources, strengths and support networks to help them identify how they would like things to be different and what is required to make this happen. Its philosophy is: 'if it ain't broke don't fix it', do more of what works and if something doesn't work, try a different approach.[22]

The counsellor collaborates with the client in finding solutions, and to do this they approach the client with a curious and open mind. The main skills used in SFT are:

- competence seeking; i.e., looking at the client's resources, skills and strengths
- asking **coping questions**, such as how the client has managed to do things in the past

- assessing motivation, via scaling questions: 'On a scale of 0 to 10 . . .'
- asking exception or discrepancy questions; that is, finding times when the problem did not exist or when it was managed better
- asking the **miracle question**: 'Imagine that while you're sleeping a miracle happens: the problem you brought here has been solved. But because you are sleeping, you don't know that this has happened. So when you wake up, what would be different to tell you that a miracle has happened and your problem is solved?'[23]

COGNITIVE BEHAVIOUR THERAPY (CBT)

Cognitive Behaviour Therapy was pioneered in the 1960s by Dr Aaron Beck, an American psychiatrist. While researching psychoanalysis, he was disappointed in findings about its effectiveness in depression. As a result he began to look for other ways of treating depression. Beck found that depressed patients experienced streams of negative thoughts that seemed to arise spontaneously, and that there were three main groups of negative thoughts: negative ideas about themselves, the world and/or the future.[24] Since that time, CBT has become one of the strongest evidence-based practices in modern-day therapy.

Cognitive Behaviour Therapy is based on the idea that cognitions affect behaviour, and that these can be changed through a range of cognitive and behavioural techniques. Cognitions refers to thoughts and underlying, often unconscious, beliefs or taken-for-granted ideas. At its essence is the idea that the way we think and what we do affects how we feel. The therapy invites the client to notice their feelings and thoughts. It is important to recognize the difference between these, as we often mix up our feelings and our thoughts, perhaps saying, 'I *feel* as though I've made a mess of things'. This is actually a thought, whereas the feeling might be sadness or disappointment. Feelings tend to be described by one word: happy, sad, angry and so on. We all have a fairly constant stream of thoughts, often automatic in nature, which can impact our feelings and behaviours.

The relationship between thinking, feeling and behaviour is shown in the CBT model in Figure 7 on the following page.

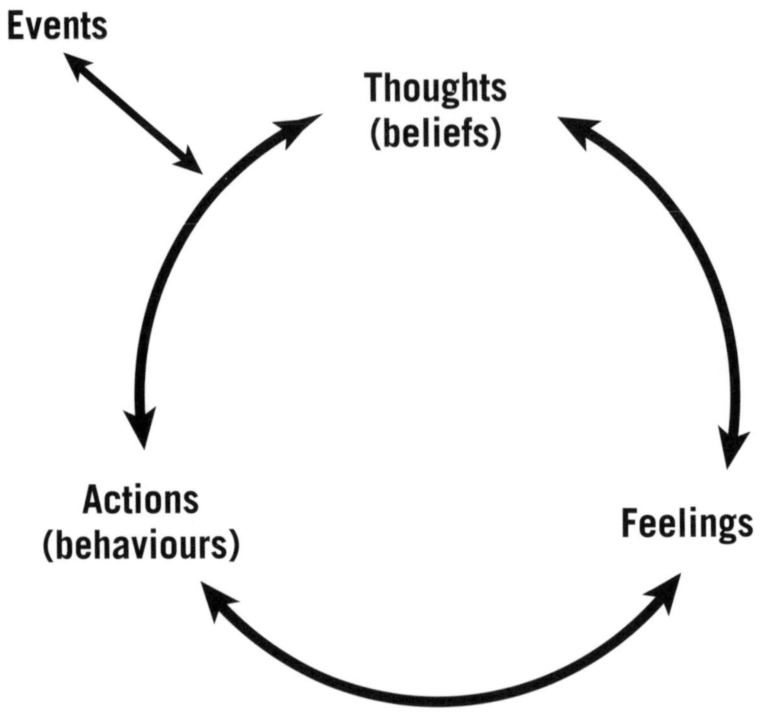

Figure 7: CBT model

The CBT model demonstrates that what you think affects how you feel, and how you feel affects what you think. And that what you do impacts on how you feel and think. Going out for a walk in nature, for example, might lift mood; focusing on everything that is going wrong will bring your mood down. Learning how thinking and feeling interact, and how to develop different ways of thinking is the basis of the cognitive part of CBT, and the role of behaviour is the basis of the behavioural part of CBT. Behavioural techniques include behavioural activation (engaging in activities), relaxation and assertiveness training. These strategies aim to break the unhelpful think–feel–do cycles, such as thinking about all that needs to be done, feeling overwhelmed and then overeating or drinking alcohol to manage that feeling.

In CBT, the counsellor works collaboratively with the client to guide them through a range of cognitive strategies. CBT teaches the client to:

- become more aware of their thinking (through thought diaries)
- recognize unhelpful thinking patterns
- challenge unhelpful thoughts
- develop more helpful ones.

Examples of unhelpful thinking patterns are shown in Table 6.

Table 6: Unhelpful thinking patterns[25]

Unhelpful thinking	Definition
All-or-nothing ('black-and-white') thinking	There is no middle ground. Things are seen in black and white; for example, if the client makes a small error at work, they see themselves as a failure.
Jumping to conclusions	The client makes a negative interpretation of things; for example, they might interpret that someone is thinking negatively about them when there is no evidence of this (called mind-reading), or they might presume that things will turn out badly.
Catastrophizing	This is overemphasizing the importance of events; a small mistake might be perceived as a disaster.
Disqualifying the positives	Discounting any positive experiences and maintaining a negative outlook.
Emotional reasoning	The client feels bad, which is seen as reflecting how things really are.
'Should' statements	The client motivates themselves with 'shoulds' and 'musts'. It is about setting high expectations, and the emotional results may be guilt, frustration or anger.
Labelling	The client uses labels, such as 'I'm a loser'.

Underlying these thinking patterns can be a range of unhelpful, often unconscious beliefs, and CBT also aims to raise awareness of these beliefs or taken-for-granted ideas and to challenge them. The following table lists a number of unhelpful beliefs; working with these will be considered in later chapters.

Table 7: Unhelpful beliefs[26]

All significant people in my life must love me and approve of me.

I must always be competent, adequate and achieving in every area of my life.

My life should progress easily and smoothly. Things should work out the way I want them to. It's awful when things go wrong.

My life experiences determine how I feel. How can I feel good when things don't go as they should?

It is better not to take risks, because when you stick your neck out, you can get easily hurt.

I must always be in control of situations.

People should be sensitive to my needs and do what I believe is right.

The world should be a fair place. I must always be treated fairly.

MINDFULNESS-BASED COGNITIVE THERAPY (MBCT)

Mindfulness-based Cognitive Therapy was developed in the 1990s by Segal, Teasdale and Williams and studied in relation to depression. It was initially designed to reduce relapse in depression. The underlying theory related to depression relapse is that individuals with a history of depression are vulnerable when their mood begins to lower, as automatic thinking patterns present during previous episodes are reactivated and can trigger onset of a new episode.[27]

MBCT challenges the fundamental CBT idea that unhelpful thinking needs to be challenged and replaced with more positive and helpful thinking. Instead, MBCT focuses on teaching individuals to become more aware of thoughts (including ruminating thought patterns) and feelings, and to relate them to a de-centred perspective as 'mental events' you can witness, rather than aspects of the self — that is, you are not your thoughts or feelings. It incorporates the practice of mindfulness and being with experience; that is, encouraging the individual to be aware of difficult thoughts and feelings, and to witness them in a different way and to foster a sense of **compassion** for yourself.

MBCT encourages the client to be more aware of thoughts and feelings and to relate to them as mental events that you can witness.

Mindfulness-based Cognitive Therapy can be taught individually by a counsellor or in an eight-week group therapy format. The initial four sessions focus on paying attention, noticing the mind wandering, and intentionally directing attention to a single, relatively neutral, focus such as the breath. The last four sessions focus on ways to skilfully handle negative mood shifts with the goal of cultivating sustained wellness.[28] Research findings from the eight-week group program have found that MBCT significantly reduces relapse rates for patients who have three or more episodes of depression. Research has also shown increased levels of mindfulness and lower levels of rumination following MBCT.[29] The skills involved in mindfulness training can increase a client's willingness to tolerate a range of internal experiences, including negative emotions.[30]

ACCEPTANCE AND COMMITMENT THERAPY (ACT)

Acceptance and Commitment Therapy was developed by American psychologist and academic, Steve Hayes. It has gained incredible momentum over the past twenty years, and there is now strong evidence that it is effective in managing anxiety, depression, eating disorders and other issues. ACT is a behavioural therapy and incorporates ideas from eastern philosophies as well as elements of a number of western therapies such as CBT, Narrative Therapy, Neuro-linguistic Programming (NLP) and Hypnotherapy. ACT receives its name from one of its central principles, namely taking action. This relates to accepting what is out of our control, and taking action that helps create a rich and meaningful life.[31]

As stated in *Release Your Worries*, 'It is important to recognize that thinking and feeling "well" does not necessarily mean that you will live a rich and meaningful life, and thinking and feeling "poorly" does not mean you can't live a rich and meaningful life'.[32] ACT proposes that the problem is struggling with anxiety-provoking thoughts and feelings, and the solution is for people to learn how to develop comfort in their own bodies and minds while still having these anxious thoughts and feelings.[33] That is, ACT advises the client to quit the struggle to think and feel better.

ACT suggests that the client focuses instead on what they can control or what they can do to live a meaningful life. The idea is for the client to become less caught up in the pain in their bodies and heads, and to get more involved in doing what they care about and value. This involves changing the relationship with the problem and developing more psychological flexibility, or being able to move between different ways of thinking and feeling. ACT encourages the acceptance of distressing emotions or events, or a willingness to experience them without trying to change them. It utilizes techniques such as cognitive defusion (including observing thoughts or thanking the mind for a thought, or singing the thought) to assist acceptance. It encourages the client to connect with the present moment (mindfulness) and to clarify and connect with their values.[34]

ACT relates to taking action to help create a rich and meaningful life. It teaches less struggle with uncomfortable feelings and thoughts, and more acceptance.

ACT encompasses the different areas or domains in life (highlighted on p. 55) and incorporates six central processes that are part of a whole:
1. Mindfulness, or contact with the present moment.
2. Defusion of feelings and thoughts.
3. Acceptance of uncomfortable feelings and thoughts and the difficult things in life.
4. Self-as-context (the part of the mind that notices thoughts and feelings, that is calm and non-judgmental).
5. Values, or living a life consistent with what is important to the client.
6. Committed action as effort and action are recognized as central to change.[35]

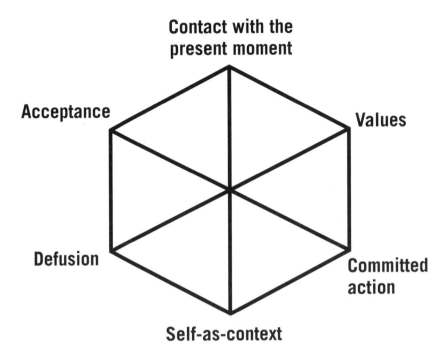

Figure 8: The ACT model

ACT provides many practical strategies to assist the client to accept and defuse uncomfortable feelings and thoughts, along with developing psychological flexibility and taking action towards a more meaningful life.

INTERPERSONAL THERAPY (IPT)

IPT was developed in the 1970s by researchers and medical psychotherapists Klerman and Weissman for the treatment of depression, and there is now good evidence that it is an effective, brief treatment for a range of mental health issues including mood disorders and eating disorders. It is based on the premise that interpersonal distress is connected with psychological symptoms, with a focus on improving interpersonal relationships. It involves interventions to reduce symptoms and improve social functioning. IPT has been adapted for use in a number of population groups, including the elderly and adolescents.

IPT recognizes the importance of the current interpersonal world in the client's symptoms and their mood, and links the mental health disorders to any relationship issues, categorizing them into four types or problem areas:

- grief due to loss
- interpersonal disputes

- role transitions (such as beginning a job, getting married)
- interpersonal sensitivities (social skills or networks).

IPT recognizes the importance of the client's interpersonal world on their symptoms, and focuses on improving interpersonal relationships.

IPT formulation

The IPT formulation is particularly helpful, and the LLCC formulation is in part based on this. The IPT formulation adopts the bio-psycho-social model, and focuses on the individual and their distress. It identifies the difficulties the individual is experiencing and categorizes them into the four types listed above. Management is then focused on these four problems areas, and there are three phases of therapy: the initial, intermediate and termination phases.[36]

Sessions in the **initial phase** involve:

- reviewing symptoms, making a diagnosis, psycho-education, reviewing the need for medication
- relating the disorder to the interpersonal context by reviewing current and past relationships as they relate to the symptoms
- identifying major problem areas and setting treatment goals, including relationship issues
- psycho-education regarding IPT concepts and processes.

Sessions in the **intermediate phase** focus on the four problem areas:

- identifying the type of grief reaction (normal, delayed, complicated) and facilitating the grieving process
- managing interpersonal disputes by choosing a plan of action, modifying unhelpful expectations or working on communication difficulties
- assisting role transitions through facilitating the grieving process and acceptance of the loss of the old role; assisting the individual to consider new roles more positively; exploring related feelings and enhancing self-belief
- addressing interpersonal sensitivities (such as shyness, impaired social skills), aiming to reduce the client's social isolation and encouraging the formation of new relationships.

Sessions in the **termination phase** involve:
- discussion about termination
- acknowledgement of grieving related to termination
- assisting the patient to recognize independent competence
- medication review and relapse prevention planning.

Management techniques for IPT come from a variety of approaches, including CBT and family systems. However, the processes of IPT focus on:
- the 'here and now'
- external relationships (rather than inner cognitions)
- resolution of relationship issues
- affect or emotions to bring about change
- the therapeutic relationship.

Key techniques in Interpersonal Therapy include:
- exploration of the client's perceptions and expectations of others
- encouragement of affect — feelings explored and expressed
- clarification of issues
- identification of problems in relationships
- problem-solving
- communication analysis (looking for incorrect assumptions and unhelpful communications) and training
- behaviour change techniques (homework such as review of old memories, e.g. photos in grief; social skills training)
- role-play
- use of the therapeutic relationship.[37]

NARRATIVE THERAPY

Narrative therapy was developed in the 1980s and 1990s by Michael White, a social worker from South Australia, and is essentially a world-view. Derived from Family Therapy, it was influenced by a number of theories and aims to bring the contents of people's lives into therapy, and to make apparent the taken-for-granted beliefs and assumptions that we make with regards to life and relationships. It is based on the idea that 'individuals construct the meaning of life in interpretive **stories**, which are then treated as "truth"' — that is, we all actively interpret our life experience and derive **meaning** that shapes our lives.[38]

Stories are made up of events, linked in sequence across time and according to plot, and they come together via language. We create stories to make sense of our lives, and these stories and their meanings have real effects on our lives. They create the lens through which we view our lives and ourselves. Multiple stories can occur at the same time, such as about our abilities, difficulties, dreams, achievements, failures, work and relationships. No single story can completely cover all aspects of the individual.[39] Some of the stories are more **dominant** and problem-saturated than others. Narrative Therapy helps clients understand these stories and to **deconstruct** the troublesome dominant stories (such as a story of neglect or trauma), and reconstruct an **alternate story** (for example, one of strength and survival).[40]

Humans are social beings, and gender, social class, culture, race and sexual orientations shape the meaning of a given situation. 'Dominant stories' imply what it means to be a person of moral worth in our culture, that is, a 'culturally' preferred way of being. We are influenced by society in relation to these stories, such as it is more attractive to be thin, and to be happy we need to be successful. We interpret the events of our lives based on how they fit with the dominant story, so that events in our lives which do not fit with the dominant story are generally not given meaning; hence, other events that take place in a person's life might not be noticed.

In addition, the person and problem tend to be seen as one and the same. For example, someone with depression may view themselves primarily as being depressed, somehow weak and to blame, rather than a competent individual who is being affected by the depression. This can result in individuals feeling helpless to make changes in their lives. The narrative approach is respectful and non-blaming, viewing problems as separate from individuals.[41]

Narrative therapy has a number of key principles, outlined below.

- The conversation between counsellor and client itself is seen as the therapy. The counsellor listens carefully and asks questions in creative ways. Reflection is used about what is happening in the conversation, leading to more effective questions and comments.
- **Curiosity** and empathy on the part of the counsellor are vital as it means we engage with the client's story and their emotions, and their understanding of those feelings. The client is encouraged to emotionally engage with their story, such as acknowledging hopes, fears and expectations.
- Circularity is another principle — that is, viewing the world as an infinite pattern of interactions.
- Everything the client says has a number of contexts, and it is important to pay attention to these.
- Conversation is a process in which two people interweave their original stories to jointly create a new one, referred to as co-creation.[42]

The narrative process aims to elicit stories that are thick and richly described.[43] The notion of metaphor is highly significant in narrative therapy, an example being the person's life as a journey and how they have overcome challenges during this journey. The aim in narrative is not to eliminate the problem, but to elicit other stories and ways of seeing the same problem. A strengths perspective is used, seeing individuals as possessing many abilities, qualities, values and skills that can assist them to change their relationship with the problem, and people are seen as the experts on themselves. The goal is to help people define what they want in life and how to use their own knowledge and skills to achieve it.

Deconstruction

Elements of the person's story may be challenged to help elicit the alternative story and to find new meanings. The process used is deconstruction of the **dominant or problem-saturated story** and reconstruction of an alternative or preferred story. It is important not to coerce the client or get ahead of them in this journey — it is the client who rewrites the story.

Deconstruction of the dominant story may involve:

- deconstructing the 'truths' the person has adopted that influence their story
- viewing the problem against cultural practices
- exploring the effects, consequences or influence of the problem in the person's life and relationships
- unravelling some of the negative conclusions the person may have reached about their identity, under the influence of the problem
- identifying power relations that people have been subject to and that have shaped their negative conclusions about their life and their identity
- more broadly redeveloping the client's strengths and resources.[44]

A technique called **externalization** can be part of deconstruction.

- Externalizing the problem or placing it outside the individual objectifies the problem as the problem, as different or distinct from the person. This is particularly important when the experience of the problem is totalizing the person's life. An example would be talking about how the problem is pushing the client around. Naming the problem or visualizing it can assist in finding new ways to take action.
- The effects of the problem in the client's life and relationships are mapped.
- Metaphors (or stories) are used, such as walking out on the problem, educating the problem, freeing life from the problem, reducing the influence of the problem or taming the problem.[45]

Reconstruction of an **alternative story** may involve the following:

- Initiate conversation and questions that will help the individual discover unique outcomes that would not have been predicted under the influence of the problem. For example, despite a traumatic childhood, the individual got through school and became a teacher to help other children. This enables what is referred to as '**re-authoring**' stories.
- Look for exceptions to the dominant story, as there are always some. Questions might explore times when the problem was not a problem for them, and what that was like.
- The client can begin to accept alternate patterns of behaviour as 'prescriptions' for who they are and may become.[46]

POSITIVE THERAPY

A relatively new field is Positive Therapy, which is based on Positive Psychology. It focuses on:

- identifying strengths and encouraging greater use of them
- fostering positive emotions including savouring, gratitude and kindness
- leisure and creativity
- engagement in life and being in 'flow' (feeling in the zone or inside the activity)
- social and emotional skills for positive relationships
- mindfulness, self-care and positive coping skills
- the role of values and authenticity
- accomplishment, purpose, meaning and hope
- resilience skills and flourishing.[47]

HYPNOTHERAPY

Hypnosis is an altered state of consciousness or a trance state, in which the client's focus of attention is concentrated.[48] It is different from sleep and different from being awake, and is similar to relaxation or meditation. It is thought to involve heightened right-brain (hemispheric) functioning, and in hypnosis the brain wave pattern changes, fluctuating between alpha (early relaxation) and delta (tranquil, creative) waves. During the day the mind regularly goes into a brief hypnotic state to relax and refresh brain function. In hypnosis, various phenomena occur such as suggestibility, time distortion (time may seem longer or shorter) and amnesia. The fact that the mind is more open to suggestion is the basis of its use as a therapy, and the hypnotherapist can assist the individual in managing thoughts, emotions or behaviours through suggestion.

Hypnotherapy is a state of focused concentration, and in hypnosis various phenomena occur, the key one being suggestibility.

There are a series of steps involved in hypnotherapy:
- pre-hypnosis (building rapport, assessment including previous experience, contraindications to hypnosis, goal-setting and education about hypnosis)
- establishing a sense of comfort and safety
- induction techniques (to focus attention)
- relaxation and deepening techniques
- teaching self-hypnosis
- direct and indirect suggestions, including metaphor
- re-alerting procedures and use of the post-hypnotic state (to reinforce suggestions used and to organize homework and follow-up)
- any take-home tasks, such as self-hypnosis or listening to recordings.

Hypnosis is said to increase the client's capacity to enhance what is already present — in other words, it can amplify their abilities. The trance state allows clients to focus on or remember positive events and memories of success, therefore reminding them what they are already capable of doing. Suggestions can also be given about achieving desired goals. As the hypnotic state is one of concentrated attention, and a relaxed and focused state is suggested, individuals can put all of their attention towards achieving their objectives. Goals are defined in the pre-hypnosis phase. Hypnotherapy can also incorporate a psychodynamic approach, utilizing the relationship with the counsellor, and access to the unconscious mind. Emotional conflicts and the meaning of events can be explored in the hypnotic state.

Hypnotherapy also assists by reducing stress and anxiety, and thereby imparting more therapeutic benefit. By being taught self-hypnosis, the client can learn to manage stress better and how to relax. Behaviours such as smoking or nail biting can be changed with hypnosis, sensations such as pain can be modified, and analgesic use can be reduced. There is a growing evidence base for the use of hypnosis in the areas of managing stress and anxiety, gastrointestinal disorders, pain management and behavioural change.[49,50] Interestingly, hypnotherapy can be used in combination with other approaches, such as MI or CBT, and research suggests that an integrated approach combining clinical hypnosis and CBT increases the efficacy of treatment.[51]

The main tool used in hypnotherapy is suggestion, and this can take several forms. Post-hypnotic suggestions are often used, such as 'Each day you will have a strong desire to exercise'. 'Ego-strengthening' (ego-S) suggestions, targeted at building confidence, are regularly used. Suggestions can also be direct or indirect. An example of a direct suggestion might be 'You are now a non-smoker' whereas an indirect suggestion might be 'You can be curious about how much you lose interest in smoking, and how that happens'.

Hypnotherapy also makes use of **metaphors** or stories, because they are part of our lives, in every culture. Stories offer us a new way to see and understand our world, and a metaphor is a therapeutic story.[52,53] Metaphors must fit the individual and the life issue. They are interactive and creative, they engage, are often indirect and contain disguised suggestions about problem-solving or behavioural change. Metaphors often explore feelings and contain meaning. They stimulate both sides of our brain (the dominant and non-dominant hemispheres), they bypass resistance to change, and they promote trance and tap the unconscious mind.[54]

LLCC TIP
Metaphors are a very useful counselling tool, and it is worth becoming skilled in using them. They are creative too!

To design a metaphor, follow these steps:
- Begin with the problem or challenge.
- Plan the metaphor and create a framework with a beginning, middle and end.
- Consider the resources you want the individual to develop and the outcome you want to achieve, and the steps required to achieve it.
- Choose any characters or symbols to be included in the metaphor, and the setting.
- Consider the layers of the metaphor, the meaning, and the feelings to be expressed.
- Consider how you can weave indirect suggestions-S through it.
- Make sure to tap into the client's senses.
- Consolidate the change and meaning at the end.[55]

To deliver a metaphor, follow these steps:

■ Tell the story so that it has life and expression.[56]
■ Pace yourself and use pauses.
■ Make your expression consistent with the story.
■ Lead the client through the story.

The following factors should be considered when deciding whether or not to use hypnosis:

■ The assessment, including personal history.
■ The presenting problem/s such as stress, anxiety, phobias, sleep problems, grief or pain, and whether hypnotherapy is an appropriate treatment for these.
■ The client's personality. For example, are they are a person who likes to be in control, and does this need to be addressed in psycho-education about hypnosis?
■ The specific objective/s for the session. Note that the assessment might take several sessions, or other treatments may need to be undertaken prior to hypnotherapy (for example, CBT).
■ Establish whether there are contraindications to the use of hypnosis such as acute psychosis, severe personality disorder, being under the age of seven, having severe depression in which concentration is low (in this case, it's best to wait until the depression is improving and then begin with relaxation). Care must be also taken if the person has dissociative episodes or has post-traumatic stress disorder.

EXPRESSIVE THERAPIES

Expressive therapies utilize the arts (such as visual arts, pottery, music, writing, drama and movement) for self-expression and enhancing personal growth. My training in expressive therapies came via OT, and short postgraduate courses in Psychodrama and Art Therapy. Expressive therapies are not a strong focus in the LLCC approach, but the use of expressive techniques is highlighted in several chapters as they can be very helpful for some clients and issues.

Expressive therapies grew from the person-centred approach of Carl Rogers and are based on the idea that all people are creative and the creative process is transformative and healing.[57] Self-awareness and insight can be fostered through expressive therapies. Art Therapy, for example, uses the creative process of making art as a safe way to explore inner experiences and raise awareness and expression.

Art Therapy

The first Art Therapy was developed by a psychoanalyst, and there are now various forms. It can provide a means for clients to express emotions that they cannot express in words. It can release information from the unconscious mind which would not otherwise be expressed. Art generated by a client can be a record of their journey in therapy, and it can be particularly helpful for young people.

Art Therapist Deborah Schroder has devised a number of applications of Art Therapy, a number of which she describes in her book, *Little Windows into Art Therapy*. They include asking the client to draw:

- what is significant in their life; the client can then decide what they want to talk about from the drawing
- their feelings, and to keep a journal of their drawings
- a visual image of their feeling, such as an 'anger monster'
- an image-filled genogram or family tree
- a 'crystal ball' with an image of what they would like life to look like; this can be repeated towards the end of counselling
- what brings them joy in life.

More recently, I undertook a series of workshops using mandalas for art therapy. Meditations were done at the start of the session about different topics, to tap into the creative and unconscious mind. Pre-drawn mandalas were used, which took the pressure off a sense of needing to draw but still enabled expression of feelings through the colours and patterns added to the templates.

BIBLIOTHERAPY

Bibliotherapy is a term used to describe using books to help people with mental and physical health problems. The goal is to broaden the client's understanding of the issues they are experiencing, and to learn ways of managing them. The client can choose to utilize Bibliotherapy as self-help, or a counsellor might recommend relevant reading as an adjunct to in-session work. Various books are recommended at the end of each chapter in this book, and a number of these can be used as self-help.

There are three types of Bibliotherapy: self-help, creative and informal. **Self-help Bibliotherapy** refers to the use of non-fiction, advisory books about different topics, to provide information and inspiration. Some are based on particular psychological approaches, such as CBT, and are often structured and manualized. This form of Bibliotherapy is quite prescriptive and there have been a number of research studies demonstrating its effectiveness.[58,59,60,61] **Creative Bibliotherapy** involves the use of fiction, poetry, biographical writing and creative writing to improve wellbeing. Such books are usually utilized with a facilitator who is familiar with the literature, but can be utilized by the client alone. **Informal Bibliotherapy** focuses on Creative Bibliotherapy techniques in an unstructured manner, including the use of reading groups or recommending texts.[62,63]

It has been known for a long time that reading can be therapeutic because of the change it can cause in the reader, about which a number of theories have been proposed. Reading creative texts can involve a psychoanalytic process, through the identification of the reader with the story, catharsis and the development of insight.[64] Cohen focused on Self-help Bibliotherapy and proposed that it developed in the reader ways of knowing and feeling.[65] Cilliers proposed three benefits: education via reading; therapy as the reader connects with characters and gains insight; and recreation.[66,67]

E-MENTAL HEALTH

Electronic or **e-mental health** refers to the use of digital technologies such as computer, phone, tablet or Internet-based programs to prevent or manage mental health issues.[68] Some programs are designed as self-help interventions and can also be used with the guidance of a counsellor. Others involve input from the therapist via phone or email. Counsellors can choose to use e-mental health in ways that suit their individual practice and the needs of the client. Based on a recent model by Reynolds and colleagues, practitioners might recommend different programs to clients, provide information about them or support the client as they utilize them. Alternatively, e-mental health might be integrated more comprehensively into sessions with clients.[69,70]

There are many advantages to e-mental health, including its convenience, efficiency, low cost and ease of access. The client is an active participant and can drive the process.[71] Generally, e-mental health programs are advised for those with mild to moderate mental health issues, and their use is dependent upon client willingness, literacy skills, vision and confidence with technology. E-mental health programs have been developed for use in the management of depression and anxiety, stress, sleep problems, chronic pain, substance use, eating disorders and body image issues.[72,73,74]

Many e-mental health treatment programs heavily utilize CBT principles. However, there are other programs that incorporate IPT, Solution-focused Therapy and Motivational Interviewing. Further information can be found in a guide on e-mental health for GPs at www.racgp.org.au.[75]

In summary

This chapter has outlined the key elements of the LLCC integrative approach, which enables you as a counsellor to consider the whole person, and to incorporate a range of approaches and therapies. The therapies utilized in the LLCC approach, such as CBT and ACT, have been introduced, and you will see their applications in different problem areas in Part 2.

Having read this chapter, consider John's story once again and how the LLCC approach may assist him, and then compare your thoughts to the ideas presented here.

Reflection on John's story

Understanding the BPSSC influences and the five Ps in John's life will be important, and drawing on a range of therapies may assist him to deal with the key issues of low mood and impact on interpersonal relationships, loss and trauma in his early years, adjusting to fatherhood and finding meaning in relation to occupation.

Exploring attachment theory and the impact of trauma may assist John to understand the impact of his early life and upbringing on his psyche and his current life. A narrative approach will bring John's story to the fore, including the history of loss and trauma, which may have resurfaced since John has had children. It will also highlight his strengths via an alternative story of coping and moving forward in life. An existential or narrative perspective will highlight the importance of meaning in John's life, in particular his love of his children and working with wood.

CBT, ACT and IPT will be helpful in working with John to improve mood. He might also benefit from Bibliotherapy and e-mental health.

Resources

Books

Corey, G. 2013, *Theory and Practice of Counseling and Psychotherapy (9th ed.)*, Cengage Learning, California.

Edelman, S. 2013, *Change Your Thinking: Positive and practical ways to overcome stress, negative emotions and self-defeating behaviour using CBT (3rd ed)*, HarperCollins Publishers, Sydney.

Egan, G. 2007, *The Skilled Helper: A problem-management and opportunity development approach to helping (8th ed.)*, Brooks/Cole Publishing, USA.

Harris, R. 2009, *ACT Made Simple: An easy-to-read primer on Acceptance and Commitment Therapy*, New Harbinger Publications, California.

Howell, C. 2010, *Keeping the Blues Away: A guide to preventing relapse of depression*, Radcliffe, London.

Howell, C. and Murphy, M., 2011, *Release Your Worries: A guide to letting go of stress and anxiety*, Exisle Publishing, New South Wales.

James, U. 2005, *Clinical Hypnosis Textbook: A guide for practical intervention*, Radcliffe, London.

Klerman, G.L., et al. 1984, *Interpersonal Psychotherapy for Depression*, Basic Books, New York.

Segal, Z.V., Williams, J.M.G. and Teasdale, J.D. 2002, *Mindfulness-based Cognitive Therapy for Depression: A new approach to preventing relapse*, The Guilford Press, New York.

Seligman, M. 2011, *Flourish: A visionary new understanding of happiness and wellbeing*, Random House Australia, Sydney.

Siegel, D.J. 2007, *The Mindful Brain: Reflection and attunement in the cultivation of wellbeing*, W.W. Norton & Company, New York.

Weissman, M., Markowitz, J. and Klerman G. 2007, *Clinician's Quick Guide to Interpersonal Psychotherapy*, Oxford University Press, Oxford.

White, M. 2007, *Maps of Narrative Practice*, W.W Norton & Company, New York.

Websites

Art Therapy: www.therapistaid.com/

CBT: www.aacbt.org

Royal Australian College of GPs, e-mental health guide: http://www.racgp.org.au/your-practice/guidelines/e-mental-health/

For information about various therapies see 'Frequently asked questions' section: www.drcatehowell.com.au

IPT: www.interpersonalpsychotherapy.org

Mindfulness and ACT: www.actmindfully.com.au

Narrative Therapy: http://dulwichcentre.com.au/

2 MANAGING LIFE ISSUES AND PROBLEM AREAS

Our anxiety does not empty tomorrow of its sorrows, but only empties today of its strengths.

—CHARLES H. SPURGEON

Part 2 is all about how you can assist the client to deal with the life issues and problem areas that they may be experiencing. Depending on where you work and the population you work with, clients will present with a range of issues and there will be some themes that emerge. I have chosen to cover some key topics which have been prominent during my working life, and which will likely to be relevant to many counsellors. These include:

- improving sleep
- managing stress and anxiety
- overcoming depression
- dealing with anger
- overcoming guilt and shame

- managing change
- loss and grief counselling
- managing trauma
- working on relationship issues
- building self-belief.

With the LLCC integrative approach, the counsellor will need to be astute and creative in their approach, asking themself which therapies and techniques are likely to best serve this client and their particular concerns, to aid their understanding, insight and skills development. The counsellor will need to take into account other factors, such as the client's age, level of intelligence and literacy, comorbidities (such as substance use disorders), personality factors or presence of any psychotic features. These factors may shape the approach to be taken (such as Motivational Interviewing being most useful in substance use disorders), or may contraindicate the use of particular therapies (such as hypnosis). In addition, the counsellor will collaborate with the client in determining which therapies to focus on. The notion of having a range of therapies to put in front of the client, to then explore and work from, enabling the client to draw from them what works best for them, can be helpful and empowering for the client.

In Part 2 you will find that with each life issue, relevant background information is provided. This information is useful for the counsellor's knowledge, but also in relation to the provision of psycho-education for the client. The therapies introduced in Part 1 are then incorporated under management, in the LLCC integrative manner. You will find ideas to assist clients based on SFT, CBT, ACT, MBCT, IPT, Narrative and Positive Therapy, expressive therapies, Hypnotherapy, Bibliotherapy and e-mental health. The LLCC approach involves working through ideas from each therapy and also using them in a more integrated way, such as reinforcing CBT or ACT via Hypnotherapy, Bibliotherapy or e-mental health, or combining aspects of therapies such as CBT and Narrative Therapy.

A suggested framework to use within each LLCC session with clients is as follows.

1. Connect with the client and do a brief mindfulness exercise.
2. Hear about the past week or two (putting on notice any issues to return to in the main part of the session).
3. Review the previous session and any take-home tasks.
4. Work on the key issues, applying the LLCC therapies and practising techniques.
5. Look at further take-home tasks and next directions.
6. Close the session.

Note that this is a guide only, though the elements of connection and mindfulness are important as they are the foundation for the remainder of the session, and ensure maximum benefit is gained. It is essential to pick up on any take-home tasks that were set, to make use of this work and to validate the client's efforts. Note that quite often the client will raise a recent event or development that needs attention. This needs to be addressed and might take up a good deal of time, but still remember the framework as a guide.

Chapter 4
Improving sleep

A well-spent day brings happy sleep.

—**LEONARDO DA VINCI**

Sleep is part of our everyday life and functioning and it is often taken for granted — until it is a problem. Unfortunately, sleep patterns can be upset by life stresses and emotional issues, such as grief, anxiety and mood disorders. Clients might find they are having trouble falling asleep or there might be a tendency to wake up in the early hours of the morning and then difficulty getting back to sleep. Some people find they sleep too much, or their sleep quality may be poor.[1]

Read the following story as an introduction to discussion about the management of sleep issues.

Marjory's story

Marjory is 85 years old and seeks help with sleep. She is finding it difficult to get off to sleep, and believes that she is only getting a few hours of sleep each night. She tells the counsellor that ideally she would like to get about 7 or 8 hours' sleep a night, and that she is becoming increasingly worried about her sleep and health as a result.

Marjory lives in a lifestyle village and enjoys socializing, reading and indoor bowls. She has heard hypnosis is useful to aid sleep. The counsellor hears more about Marjory, completes the assessment and begins to think about what approaches might assist her.

Background

Sufficient sleep is vital to maintaining physical and mental health. The length of sleep deemed sufficient will depend on your age and individual variations, but 8 hours is a general recommendation.[2] Our sleep patterns are regulated by our **circadian rhythm**, which is based on light. In the evening, when the sun goes down, our brain releases hormones that make us sleepy. In the morning, daylight triggers the release of different hormones that will keep us awake.[3] Normally, our circadian rhythm and sleep balance are aligned, but travel or shift work can disrupt these.[4] Prolonged disruption of these systems is detrimental to health.[5]

There are two types of sleep: non-rapid eye movement (NREM) and rapid eye movement (REM). Each phase of NREM sleep lasts 90 to 120 minutes and contributes to restoration and growth of the body, and this will vary with age. In contrast, REM sleep plays a key role in learning and memory. REM sleep occurs three to five times per night, taking up 90 to 120 minutes, with most REM sleep occurring in the morning hours.[6] Older adults spend less time in REM sleep than younger people.[7]

During sleep, our body cycles through five different stages, each with varied levels of brain activity.[8] Most people experience four to six cycles per night.[9]

Table 8: The sleep cycle[10]

Type of sleep	Cycle	What happens during this cycle
NREM sleep	1	Dozing or drowsiness
	2	Light sleep. Body temperature drops, breathing and heart rate slow
	3 & 4	Deep sleep. Low blood pressure, slow heart rate and breathing. Muscles relaxed. Important stage for body growth/repair. Slow brain waves.
REM sleep	5	Eyes jerk under lids. Brain activity similar to waking. Heart rate, blood pressure and breathing rate rise. Limbs paralyzed. Most dreaming occurs in REM sleep.

Poor sleep is common and can be due to shift work or travel, issues such as stress, anxiety or depression, drug or alcohol misuse, too much caffeine or nicotine, sleep apnoea or poor sleeping habits (e.g. being on the Internet late into the night). Short-term sleep deprivation can adversely affect concentration, memory, mood and judgment, as well as decision making, reaction time and physical coordination. It can also increase the risk of accidents.[11] In the long term, sleep deprivation correlates with obesity, diabetes, mood disorders, cardiovascular disease and even early mortality.[12]

LLCC management

Management begins with an appropriate assessment, which includes hearing the client's story and ensuring medical causes for sleep problems (such as sleep apnoea) have been ruled out by the client's GP. **Psycho-education** is a key management tool in dealing with sleep difficulties. It is helpful to talk with clients about the nature of sleep, to aid understanding, as sometimes there are unrealistic expectations about sleep. There are many strategies that can improve sleep patterns. We will draw on ideas from **CBT**, **ACT** and **Hypnotherapy**. It is important to recognize that it takes time for sleep to improve, so patience and consistency in applying the strategies are necessary.

The table on the following page summarizes common causes of poor sleep and the various management options.

Table 9: Common causes of sleep problems and management[13]

Common cause	Options
Daytime naps	Restrict sleep to the evenings.
Too much rest during day	Try to keep physically and mentally active through the day.
Worry, stress	Deal with worries before bed, use relaxation techniques and mental distractions. The client might need to get up and repeat their sleep wind down, or do a calming activity until they feel ready for sleep.
Medication misuse or withdrawal	It might take a few days to a week for various medications to be out of the body. These effects will pass in time. It is advisable to work with a GP when withdrawing from medication.
Stimulants before bed	Stop drinking tea/coffee in the evening. Replace with warm, caffeine-free drinks such as herbal teas or milk.
Pain/discomfort	Pace activities during the day. Pain can be worse at night because there are fewer distractions — use relaxation techniques and distracting imagery.
Alcohol in the evening	Avoid or limit the amount.
Depression, anxiety	Appropriate psychological treatment and/or medication.
Trying too hard to sleep — tossing and turning	Relaxation techniques. Get up and do something calming. Might need to repeat several times.
Late-night activities that get your brain racing	Avoid these activities in the evening. Plan for more relaxing, pleasant tasks before bed.
Going to bed at irregular hours or often sleeping late in the mornings	Establish a regular routine, and avoid TV, computers or reading in bed. Get up at the same time each day.

The **CBT** approach involves keeping records. Keeping a **sleep diary** is a good place to start when working on sleep issues. This involves keeping a record of activities and sleeping patterns for a week or so, to help identify where the client is having trouble and whether there is any pattern. Ask the client to fill in their sleep diary for the full 24 hours, and keep it for at least a few days. This will enable you to work out the best way to deal with the problems. It helps to advise the client to keep it beside their bed and to fill it in each morning.

Table 10: Sample sleep diary[14]

Time of day	Activity	Sleep
7 p.m.	Dinner	
8 p.m.	TV	
9 p.m.	Cup of tea	
10 p.m.		Nap in lounge chair
11 p.m.		
12 midnight		Off to sleep
1 a.m.		
2 a.m.		Woke up

Sleep hygiene

Once the sleep issues have been established, it is useful to help the client utilize a range of behavioural strategies to aid sleep. This is called sleep hygiene. It can be helpful to talk through the various recommendations with the client and see which are relevant to the individual.

The main points to discuss in terms of sleep hygiene are as follows:

- Reduce demands in life; be aware of tiredness and the need for rest.
- Re-establish a sleep routine, that is, go to bed at about the same time each night and get up at the same time each morning.
- Develop a bedtime ritual, for example: hot milk drink, teeth and toilet, then bed.
- Bed is a place for sleeping and intimacy — not doing work or watching television.
- Make sure the bed and pillows are comfortable, and the bedroom is dark and a comfortable temperature.
- Some people find that a couple of drops of an essential oil (such as lavender) on the pillow is soothing, though advise the client to check first that they are not overly sensitive to the smell or allergic to the oil.
- Turn the alarm clock away so there is no temptation to watch it.[15]
- Have a wind-down or relaxation time before going to bed. For example, enjoy a warm bath a good hour or two before bed, read for a while or listen to peaceful music.
- Use relaxation techniques and meditation (recordings are often helpful) before sleep or if wakeful during the night (a range of techniques are described later in this chapter).

Encourage the client to utilize a range of behavioural strategies, or sleep hygiene, to aid sleep. For example, relaxation techniques or meditation.

- If awake for over 30 minutes during the night, it is best to get up and repeat the wind-down routine.
- If not sleeping well at night, it is best to avoid sleeping during the day or dozing off in the chair in the evening.
- Manage stress, so that the mind is more peaceful when retiring.
- If something is worrying the client at night, it is best to write it down so they can deal with it the next day. Encourage them to keep a pen and paper next to the bed.
- Exercise during the day to then be more physically tired at night (avoid exercising heavily just before bed, as this tends to raise alertness).
- Take a walk in the early morning sunlight, preferably without sunglasses. When sunlight enters the eye, it helps to regulate the body's natural sleep–wake cycle; it also stimulates the production of serotonin, which can assist in mood regulation.
- Avoid too much caffeine or alcohol, as both can disturb sleep.
- Avoid overeating in the evening. On the other hand, having a light supper (for example, a banana and a milk drink) can aid sleep.
- Avoid using computers or other screens for at least an hour before bed, as the blue light they emit interferes with melatonin secretion (the hormone that prepares the body for sleep). You can download an application called 'f.lux', which matches the light from your computer to the light of the room you're in (see https://justgetflux.com/).[16,17]

A behavioural technique attracting attention is **sleep restriction**. When there has been insomnia, the bed can become a place of distress and arousal. A diary is kept to determine the average amount of sleep the client is having over a week. There is an assumption made that clients tend to underestimate the sleep they obtain, hence the time in bed is restricted and sleep is therefore also restricted. Over several nights the quality of sleep can improve significantly. The length of time in bed is gradually increased by 15 minutes at a time. This technique is best used by counsellors trained in this technique to ensure safety.[18]

CBT techniques also involve addressing worrying thoughts that might be deterring sleep, or worries about finding it difficult to sleep. Remind the client that even if not actually asleep, resting and relaxing are still beneficial to the mind and body. Strategies from CBT to identify and challenge unhelpful thinking, or from ACT to defuse worrying thoughts, can also assist. This involves working on acceptance that sleep will be disturbed for a while, and fostering the client's thinking that they are doing the best they can and that their sleep will improve over time. Two examples follow.

1. The client looks at the clock every 30 minutes and thinks; 'I will never get to sleep, this is terrible. I need to sleep to be able to work properly tomorrow.' Using CBT, a more helpful series of thoughts might be encouraged, such as: 'Turn the clock around, just rest and relax and sleep will follow. It will be okay.'

2. The clients thinks 'Why can't I sleep? I can't believe this, I have to get some rest.' Using ACT the thinking can be changed to: 'I am having the thought "Why can't I sleep?" Thank you brain,' and then the client visualizes putting these thoughts on a cloud and letting them float off, or onto leaves and letting them drift away down a stream.

Strategies from CBT to identify and challenge unhelpful thinking, or from ACT to defuse worrying thoughts, can assist sleep. Hypnotherapy can also be utilized in a variety of ways to aid sleep.

Hypnotherapy

The use of hypnotherapy to aid sleep is well established, and it can be utilized in a variety of ways to improve disturbed sleeping patterns. The relaxation in hypnosis is useful in itself, as is self-hypnosis.[19] Individuals can engage in hypnotherapy to relax their mind and body, and this can ease them into falling asleep; others just daydream in their safe space in a trance, waiting for sleep to come.

Hypnotherapy to assist sleep involves:

- assessment, followed by **education** about sleep hygiene and hypnosis
- induction, deepening, and teaching **self-hypnosis**
- **direct suggestions** re: sleep, begin **sleep strategies**
- suggestions regarding progress (ego-S), further sleep strategies
- review progress each session, reinforce suggestions, possibly using metaphor (for example, holiday, active and relaxed, sleep well . . .).

Following are the steps for teaching self-hypnosis to aid sleep (note that these steps can be adapted when teaching self-hypnosis to assist any issue):

1. Suggest that it is useful to use self-hypnosis both for relaxation and to put into action a number of sleep techniques.
2. Suggest the client makes time for self-hypnosis in bed. It can be used before sleep and they can drift off to sleep following self-hypnosis.
3. Suggest that there is always part of the mind looking after the individual (the 'hidden observer'), and that the client will become alert again if there is something important for them to attend to.
4. Let the client know to adjust both the lighting and temperature in the bedroom, then make themselves comfortable in the bed.
5. Following an induction, the hypnosis is deepened via muscle relaxation, breathing, counting down to a special place . . . let the client know to enjoy the relaxation then use the sleep techniques (below).

The specific sleep techniques I have found most helpful for clients are adapted from sleep scripts by Hunter.[20] You might not be trained in hypnosis. However, these scripts still can be used to build on relaxation training.

Imagine a whiteboard in your mind. You have a whiteboard marker and a cloth. In the top left-hand corner, slowly write number one — tap into how you feel and look as you do this. Then in the middle of the board slowly write a word to do with sleep [such as pillow]. Look at the word. Then slowly rub the number one and your first word out. Now write number two in the top right-hand corner of the board, and another word to do with sleep in the middle of the board. Slowly rub them out. Then write the number three in the bottom right-hand corner of the board, and another word to do with sleep in the centre. Again, rub them out. Next, write number four in the bottom left-hand corner of the board. Write another word to do with sleep in the centre of the board. Slowly rub these out, and then continue on. You might be surprised about how few numbers and words you actually write before sleep comes.

Count slowly backwards from 300 in your mind. If the numbers become confused, just restart around that number and continue on.

Make as many words as you can out of the letters of the word Constantinople.

Imagine wandering along a pathway that has a number of other little paths going off from it [or you can use a corridor with rooms off it]. You wander along slowly, feeling peaceful and safe, and decide to explore some of the side paths. You find that each of them has something to do with sleep; one might lead to a spot with two shady trees and a comfortable hammock, another might lead to a comfy bed with clean sheets and lovely pillows, and yet another might lead to a warm bath. Take your time and enjoy each one, feeling more and more relaxed and sleepy as you do.

In summary

Clients frequently complain of sleep issues, especially when anxiety or depression symptoms are present. Sleep can also be disturbed during stressful times and during grief. It is therefore essential to have a good understanding of sleep issues and to be able to take clients through a range of strategies to improve sleep.

Reflection on Marjory's story

The counsellor connected well with Marjory, and could sense her struggle with her perception about not getting enough sleep. She began by providing psycho-education about sleep, including information about the number of hours of sleep potentially declining as we get older. The counsellor also encouraged helpful patterns of behaviour in relation to sleep, and taught Marjory relaxation techniques and self-hypnosis. Marjory adopted the ideas enthusiastically. She found these techniques helped her relax and to be more accepting of her sleep patterns. She found that her worry lessened and she sensed some improvement in sleep.

LLCC TIPS: TO AID SLEEP

Ask your client to follow these ten steps for improved sleep.

- Keep a sleep diary.
- Re-establish a sleep routine and bedtime ritual.
- Turn off any screens (computer, tablet, phone, TV) one hour before sleep.
- Use relaxation techniques.
- Try some hypnotic techniques.
- Avoid sleep during the day.
- Manage stress.
- Create a comfortable bedroom.
- Exercise during the day.
- Avoid too much caffeine or alcohol.

Resources

Websites

Healthy Sleep: http://healthysleep.med.harvard.edu/interactive/circadian

Sleep Health Foundation: http://www.sleephealthfoundation.org.au

Centre for Clinical Interventions: http://www.cci.health.wa.gov.au

Better Health Channel fact sheet — sleep: http://www.betterhealth.vic.gov.au/bhcv2/bhcarticles.nsf/pages/sleep

Better Health Channel fact sheet — sleep hygiene: http://www.betterhealth.vic.gov.au/bhcv2/bhcarticles.nsf/pages/Sleep_hygiene?open

Australian Centre for Education in Sleep: www.sleepeducation.net.au/publications.php

Phone apps

Take a Break guided meditations

iSleep Easy meditations for sleep

Smiling Mind: www.smilingmind.com.au

Meditation Oasis: www.meditationoasis.com/apps/

Chapter 5
Managing stress and anxiety

The greatest weapon against stress is the ability to choose one thought over another.

—WILLIAM JAMES

Stress and anxiety are part of life, and clients commonly present to the counselling setting with high levels of stress and symptoms of anxiety. Stress is defined as a response to a demand which is being experienced, and it can occur when responding to an issue at work, when out socially or planning a social occasion, or at home when renovating or experiencing conflict, for example. Stress can result from positive events, such as planning a wedding, and can also result from the many demands placed on us in the modern world, including technology and multi-tasking. Stress can be helpful and spur an individual on to achieve things, but unfortunately stress can also impact on quality of life and health. Stress is an individual experience and has different meanings for different people. Some people might describe stress as tension, others as worry, or feeling overwhelmed, or out of control.[1]

Read the following story and then as you go through the chapter, reflect on the nature of the stress affecting Bill, and which approaches might assist him.

Bill's story

Bill is a 39-year-old married man who works as a manager at an advertising firm. When the counsellor explores Bill's concerns, Bill explains that he is fed up with feeling worried all the time, and that there is always something in his mind that creates worry. He reports that he has felt worried like this for about 12 months. In the past two years, there have been major life changes — a job change, moving house and the birth of his third child. Bill is also having difficulty sleeping, and has had a number of panic attacks since a recent interstate trip for work. There is a family history of Bipolar Disorder, and he is fearful of having this. He is drinking around two to three shots of scotch each night to assist sleep.

Background

Anxiety is a normal and universal emotion, and is related to one of our key emotions, fear. We all know the feeling of fear, whether related to a job interview, giving a talk or a fear of heights. There are some similarities between excitement and anxiety. We can recognize when we are feeling frightened or anxious by what we experience in our mind and body. These responses can help us survive in a dangerous situation, but in many cases anxiety can be distressing and can significantly interfere with a person's home life, relationships or work. Anxiety is typically about something that might happen in the future. When a person feels anxious, they might be anticipating a problem or there might actually be some element of danger, such as when driving on a busy freeway.[2,3]

LLCC TIP

Anxiety is typically about something that might happen in the future. Listen out for the words 'what if'. For example, 'What if I lose my job?' or 'What if I have [a particular] disease?'

The therapeutic approaches to managing stress and anxiety are similar. However, it is important to differentiate stress and anxiety from experiencing an **anxiety disorder**. When anxiety is excessive or interferes with the person's ability to lead their life, such as their ability to work or attend social functions, it becomes a problem and might fit with being an anxiety disorder. One of the reasons for identifying such disorders is that, although similar principles apply in management, specific approaches may be used with the different anxiety disorders. A comprehensive assessment will assist, or you might want to collaborate with other professionals to assist with identifying a particular anxiety disorder.

When anxiety symptoms are distressing and interfere with the person's ability to carry out their daily activities, this is referred to as an anxiety disorder. Similar management principles might apply, but it is important to be aware that specific treatments may be needed.

A number of anxiety disorders have been identified, including the following.

- Generalized Anxiety Disorder (GAD) or worrying most days for over 6 months. The client might say they have always been a worrier. People who experience GAD are pushed around by the belief that they can do little to predict and control events in life, so they end up worrying about them. However, worrying can be unproductive as it often stops people engaging in activity and in problem-solving.[4]
- Specific phobias. With specific phobias, an individual has an unrelenting and irrational fear of a specific object or situation, such as a fear of enclosed spaces (claustrophobia) or a fear related to an animal or heights. This fear usually leads to avoidance of the object or situation.
- Social Anxiety Disorder (SAD) is the fear of being negatively evaluated by others or being embarrassed. Performance anxiety is a form of Social Anxiety Disorder.
- Panic Disorder involves repeated discrete episodes of severe anxiety, often 'out of the blue', with worry about having further episodes.
- Agoraphobia is another anxiety disorder and can be associated with

panic disorder. With agoraphobia, the individual becomes anxious about being in a situation in which it might be difficult to escape or which could be embarrassing. It often leads to avoidance of the feared situations, such as crowded places, buses or shopping centres.

- Obsessive-compulsive Disorder (OCD) involves ruminating about particular fears and carrying out compulsive behaviours with the aim of relieving the anxiety.
- Post-traumatic Stress Disorder (PTSD) and Acute Stress Disorder sit in their own category related to experiencing trauma beyond our normal experience, in which our own life or the lives of others are threatened.
- Some clients experience excessive worry about their health, often ruminating on having serious a diagnosis such as cancer. This is referred to as health anxiety or Somatic Symptom Disorder.[5]

LLCC management

With anxiety, it is vital to do a comprehensive assessment as outlined in Part 1, including a formulation and the preparation of a management plan. It can be helpful to prioritize the issues of concern with the client and set some goals collaboratively. It is always worth reflecting with the client on whether stress or anxiety has occurred before, and what has helped the client manage previously. Often, using these strategies again can be helpful. When a client is feeling stressed or anxious, it is helpful to be supportive and reassuring, and to focus at the start on providing **psycho-education**, such as discussion about the physiology of anxiety (the fight or flight response), the range of symptoms in anxiety, the common myths, as well as lifestyle measures which can assist.

Psycho-education about the potential management approaches is also helpful, such as about **SFT**, **CBT**, **IPT**, **Narrative Therapy** or **Hypnotherapy** (refer to the summaries in Chapter 3). The counsellor explains the therapies they are going to utilize. Remember, too, that there are also some very useful **self-help books** and **e-mental health** programs to draw on as well.

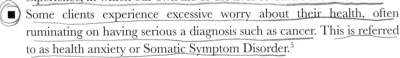

Be supportive and reassuring, and focus at the start on providing psycho-education, including potential management approaches. Don't forget relevant self-help books and e-mental health programs.

At the core of all anxiety is the body's stress or **fight or flight response**. An important aspect of psycho-education for all clients with anxiety is explaining this response to the client, and a useful summary of this response is adapted here from *Release Your Worries*. When an individual is under stress or threat, the mind and body will react with the fight or flight response. This response is, in fact, designed to protect us rather than harm us. In the age of the 'caveman', an everyday danger might have been coming face to face with a dangerous animal, such as a sabre-toothed tiger, when out hunting for food. The caveman would have been fearful of the tiger, which would have been able to kill him. In this scenario, the caveman would have seen the tiger in his path, recognized the danger, and then a number of changes would have automatically happened in his body and mind. These changes would have included:

- a change in blood flow to prepare the body for activity; There would have been a redirection of blood flow from the brain, skin and extremities (fingers, toes), the intestines and other organs to the muscles, so that the caveman could either run away or fight the tiger
- the movement of glucose from stores in the body into the blood to provide energy
- an increase in alertness through the senses (hearing, sight, smell)
- an increase in sweating to cool the body and make the skin slippery
- a reduction in saliva production
- a reduction in other body functions, such as digestion
- an increase in heart rate to pump blood to necessary parts of the body
- an increase in breathing rate to get more oxygen into the body.[6]

The same changes still happen in the mind and body when there is any significant stress or threat. This might not be a wild animal in today's world, but it could be a job redundancy, an interpersonal conflict or a divorce dispute. The physical changes that accompany stress are intense but tend to be of limited duration. When we are in danger, the brain is generally stimulated, causing an increased nervousness and alertness. The hypothalamus and pituitary gland in the brain are also stimulated and trigger an increase in activity in the sympathetic nervous system, which controls functions such as heart rate, breathing rate, blood pressure and sweating. The stress response also activates the adrenal glands, which release a number of hormones, including adrenaline, into the bloodstream. These hormones also increase the sympathetic nervous system effects. This is why we might experience rapid breathing, a racing heart or palpitations when we are stressed or anxious, or feeling hyper-alert.[7]

These changes result in the various symptoms experienced in stress and anxiety, summarized in Table 11.

Table 11: Symptoms of stress and anxiety[8]

Physical	Emotional	Cognitive	Behavioural	Social
Headaches	Feeling tense, anxious	Negative thoughts	Changes in eating, smoking or alcohol use	Inability to fulfill social roles
Tiredness	Irritability or anger	Thoughts about not being able to cope	Problems managing time	Impact on relationships at home or work
Sleeping problems	Overly sensitive/ reactive	Poor concentration	Rushing things, having mishaps	
Muscle tightness or cramps	Feeling low in mood		Nail biting	Visiting doctor frequently
Teeth grinding	Low motivation	Impaired decision-making	Avoiding different situations	
Dizziness	Fear of being embarrassed socially			
Breathlessness		Forgetfulness	Lowered libido	
Palpitations		Bad dreams		
Chest discomfort	Fear of having a serious illness			
Diarrhoea				

There are many misconceptions about anxiety, and it is important to also talk to clients about some of these common myths.[9] You might want to discuss the following myths, in bold, followed by the reality:

- **'Anxiety isn't real.'** The fight or flight response is very real.
- **'Anxiety can be harmful.'** Although the symptoms are uncomfortable, anxiety will generally not harm the individual.
- **'I'll have a heart attack.'** Anxiety does not generally impact adversely on the heart.
- **'I'll lose control.'** The person might feel very distressed and agitated, or might withdraw, but will not 'lose control'.
- **'I'll go crazy.'** Anxiety can be distressing and sometimes cause the person to feel dissociated (separate from) their body, for example, but they do not lose touch with reality.
- **'I'll faint.'** The shallow breathing in anxiety can trigger dizziness or faint feelings, but it is very unusual to faint from anxiety.
- **'Anxiety is a sign of weakness.'** Anxiety is part of life and, in fact, it takes great courage to deal with anxiety.

Addressing lifestyle is also important in managing stress and anxiety. Consider the following questions with the client:

LLCC TIP

Suggest to the client to have a pen and paper by the bed, and jot down any thoughts before turning off the light. These thoughts can be dealt with the next day, hence, there is no need to ruminate any more on them.

- Is the client able to sleep and getting enough sleep? Sleep can be affected in stress and anxiety, and using the sleep education and hygiene strategies covered in Chapter 4 can be very helpful for the client.
- Are they eating regularly and fairly healthily? Encourage sound nutrition.
- Do they undertake some exercise, or could they begin some regular walking, yoga or tai chi? Exercise can help clients to unwind and release some of the stress.
- Are there any substances aggravating their symptoms, such as nicotine, caffeine or amphetamines? Does use of these need to be addressed?
- Do they make time to relax regularly? Relaxation can be different things to different people, so it is useful to explore what activities they find relaxing — whether reading a book, listening to music or doing some exercise, for example — and encourage these.
- Do they prioritize themselves and practise self-care, including saying 'no' some of the time?
- Are they doing activities they value in life, having social contact with family and friends, or having a laugh regularly?

When there is stress or anxiety it is vital to address lifestyle — sleep, eating, exercise, reducing any substance use, regular relaxation, self-care and engaging in enjoyable activities.

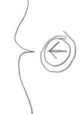

A very useful psycho-education tool is a metaphor called the **stress bucket**. Every day of our lives is filled with demands, from getting up in the morning, to doing things for family members, going to work and paying bills. If the client imagines themselves as a bucket with a finite capacity for stress, and then imagines that every demand made upon them is a drop of stress in their bucket, it is easy to imagine how the bucket can fill and overflow when demands build up. They might find that they 'spill over' with emotions and behaviours that are not usual for them.[10] Some people will have more stress in their bucket than others because of their lifestyle, life circumstances, personality and how they view the world. However, there is something that the client can do to lower the level of stress in their bucket — **relaxation**, as this is the opposite of the stress response. Due to the ongoing nature of stress in modern life the client may have become disconnected with their relaxation response and need to relearn it.

LLCC TIP

Consider having a picture of a bucket or a real bucket in your office, or alternatively draw a bucket on a piece of paper or whiteboard. This will aid you in explaining the stress bucket metaphor.

The advantage of a real bucket is that you can place in it a few props related to stress-reduction strategies, such as a relaxation CD, a book, a music CD, a picture of someone walking on the beach . . . to bring discussion about this to life.

Breathing techniques

In the first sessions with a client experiencing stress or anxiety, it is beneficial to guide them through some breathing techniques. This will give them a tool to use immediately, and give them a sense that they are able to begin to tame the anxiety. Guide the client to count their breathing over 30 seconds (a breath in and a breath out is one breath). A person feeling calm takes about ten to twelve breaths a minute, but during stress or anxiety the rate can climb to 25 breaths a minute. I often say that I will count my breath at the same time, to reduce the client feeling self-conscious. Say 'start' when you start timing and 'stop' once the 30 seconds is up. You then double the count to get the breathing rate over 1 minute.

LLCC TIP

In the first sessions with the client, it is beneficial to guide them through some breathing techniques that they can begin to use immediately.

I will often frame discussion about learning some techniques to breathe effectively in this way:

> *A good skill to begin with is breathing. When experiencing stress and anxiety, our breathing rates can alter, often increasing, and breaths can become shallow. The usual resting breathing rate in an adult is about twelve breaths per minute, but when anxious this can go up to 25 breaths per minute. People commonly report a sense of breathlessness, especially when experiencing panic. Breathing skills can help you feel calmer and more relaxed, and can help prevent some of the other physical anxiety symptoms from developing, such as dizziness. So why don't we go through a few different techniques and you can then choose one that fits best for you.*

It is also important to explain to clients that they need to set aside some time to use their new breathing exercises, maybe each day or several times a day. This is because, as with everything we learn, practice is essential. You might choose to encourage them to keep a record of their practice for a week or two. Here are a few breathing techniques that may be helpful for your clients.

SLOW BREATHING

> *The larger volumes of the lungs are at the base of the lungs, and so effective breathing means expanding the chest by lowering the diaphragm. In doing so, the abdomen moves outwards. Often we think taking a full breath involves raising the shoulders, but this is not the case as this is where the smaller volumes of the lungs are.*
>
> *Place your hands just below your diaphragm with the fingers of each hand lightly touching those of the other, and then take medium-sized breaths and focus on breathing down into your abdomen. You will find that your fingers move slightly apart. Aim to breathe in for three counts and out for three counts — counting in, two, three and out, two, three — and this this will lead to you taking about ten to twelve breaths a minute. Sometimes it can be helpful to imagine that the abdomen is like a balloon, and when you breathe in you fill the balloon.*

AWARENESS OF THE BREATH

> *Breathe in and out through your nose if comfortable with this, or in through the nose and out through the mouth. Simply be aware of the breath in and then the breath out. Breathe at a gentle, slow pace, and feel the cooler air moving in. Breathe out and feel the warmer air move out. Repeat several times.*
>
> *You might like to incorporate saying 'relax', 'peace' or 'calm' in your mind as you breathe out, and focus on letting go of tension and stress each time you breathe out.[11]*

MINDFUL BREATHING

Observe and feel the breath. Rest your attention on where the air enters and leaves the body, whether that be through the nose or the mouth. Maintain your focus on this for a few minutes.

During this exercise, distracting thoughts or images might come into your mind. There is no need to try to stop these thoughts coming into the mind. Simply notice them, and let them pass, allowing the attention to return gently to an awareness of the breath.[12]

COUNTING THE BREATH

Count 'one' on your first in-breath and 'one' on your first out-breath, then 'two' on the next in-breath and 'two' on the next out-breath, and so on. Keep doing this until you reach ten then start again at one. Or you might want to note the 'in' and the 'out' of the breath itself — think 'in' as you breathe in, and 'out' as you breathe out.[13]

COGNITIVE BEHAVIOUR THERAPY

CBT involves cognitive and behavioural strategies. Breathing techniques fall under CBT, as they are behavioural techniques. You might want to explore other relaxation techniques with the client, such as progressive muscle relaxation and visualization, as relaxation is the body's own way of recovering from stress and anxiety. Sometimes individuals lose touch with this natural response due to the demands they have on them. However, relaxation can be relearned with some effort. Relaxation is a way of producing a calm body and a quiet mind, and clients can lower the level of stress in their bucket by regular relaxation practice. In this way it is a preventive activity, and it is important to encourage its use in this way.

When teaching relaxation to a client for the first time, have them sitting in a chair because this position is easy to adapt to everyday life. For example, they can then use the relaxation techniques while sitting at their desk at work or while sitting in a shopping centre or on a bus. The relaxation position also involves having feet flat on the floor and hands resting on the thighs. Below are some guidelines to share with the client to help them prepare for relaxation.

- Do not do relaxation directly after strenuous exercise, or after a big meal.
- Ensure you go to the toilet before starting relaxation.
- Try to ensure there will be no interruptions by taking the phone off the hook, turning off other phones, informing others about not being available for a while, or putting a 'do not disturb' sign on the door.
- Make sure the room is not too hot or too cold, and turn down the lights.
- Consider removing contact lenses or glasses and wear comfortable, loose clothing.[14]

LLCC TIP

There are some cautions with relaxation. The following individuals might find relaxation techniques difficult or unhelpful:

- people who dissociate readily, or those with active psychotic symptoms
- those with severe depression (as concentration might be limited).

There are many different relaxation techniques but primarily, techniques can be physical or mental or a combination of both. Different clients will be able to relax in different ways; some might relax through visual means, such as reading, movies, or enjoying looking at the ocean; some might relax through the 'auditory' sense or sound, such as nature sounds or music; and others might like to relax through the 'kinesthetic' sense or movement, such as walking, swimming or tai chi. What follows are two relaxation scripts which you might find helpful with your clients. The first is a progressive muscle relaxation, and the second is one that taps into the senses. Once you have explained relaxation and its use, you can offer to talk the client through scripts such as these. Remember to gain consent from the client to do so, and to speak slowly and calmly as you take them through the relaxation, and monitor them as you go. See 'Resources' at end of the chapter for quality recordings or phone apps fo relaxation.

PROGRESSIVE MUSCLE RELAXATION

Make yourself comfortable and allow your eyes to close or focus on a spot in front of you. Be aware of your feet on the floor and hands on your lap. Breathe gently in and out at a medium rate. As we go through the different parts of the body, notice how the muscles in that area are feeling. You may pick up some tightness or tension. But as you learn to let go of tension in the muscles, they will loosen and feel more comfortable.

To begin with, focus on the muscles in the face and notice how they feel. You might want to move them to get a sense of that. Then allow the muscles in the forehead to loosen and relax . . . and the muscles around the eyes, into the cheeks and the jaw. Let the teeth sit a little apart. Now allow the scalp to loosen and relax, and the neck muscles, particularly the muscles at the back of the neck. Let the shoulder muscles loosen and relax . . . and now let relaxation flow down through the upper arms, forearms and into the hands, any tension leaving through the fingertips.

Be aware of your breath again, and the gentle movements of your chest with your breathing. Notice the chest muscles relaxing with each breath, and feel the abdomen move with your breath, and relax. Allow the back muscles to relax from the top of the spine to the base of the spine, the buttock muscles relaxing too. Then allow relaxation to flow down through the thighs, down through the calves, and down into the feet and toes, any tension flowing out through the toes.

Enjoy greater feelings of relaxation from head to toe, and you can return your focus of attention to any part of the body that needs a little bit more time to loosen and relax. Then, when you are ready, have a gentle stretch, and gradually open your eyes to bring your attention back to the room.

SENSORY RELAXATION

This script will allow the client to become more aware of which senses they feel more comfortable with. It is important to let them know not to be concerned if they can't visualize very well, but instead they can focus on one of the other senses they relate to better.

Sit comfortably and allow your eyes to close. Relax more deeply as you imagine a path that leads down to the front gate of a two-story cottage. Feel the path under your feet and the sunshine on your face. There is a wooden gate that opens into a pretty cottage garden with flowers on either side of the path. Notice what you can see, hear, touch or smell in the garden.

Then enter the house through the blue front door. It leads into a welcoming entrance hall with a hallstand. Do you feel the house welcoming you? There is a room on the left, a sitting room with a comfortable lounge with striped upholstery, with light coming through the window. Notice all that you can see in the room and how comfortable the lounge looks. There is another room on the other side of the hall. It has a stereo with all the music that you like available — you can sit there to listen to and enjoy the music. When you are finished there, make your way to the kitchen. There is the smell of delicious cooking — what's in the oven? Take some time to smell and taste the food.

Up a small staircase there is a bedroom with a comfortable bed, a thick quilt and lovely pillows to lie down on and have a rest. How does it feel to lie there? Is it incredibly comfortable?

When you are ready, return downstairs and explore the garden if you would like to. There are many plants and flowers and corners of the garden to explore. There is also a surprise for you in one corner — maybe a lovely fountain or a favourite flower. Enjoy the cottage and garden for a few moments more and, when you're ready, come back to the here and now.[15]

AVOIDANCE

The concept of avoidance in anxiety was mentioned earlier. As anxiety is related to fear, the client will often react by avoiding situations in which fear arises — for example, if there is a fear of using an escalator, they might take the stairs instead. Excessive avoidance is responsible for turning anxieties into life-limiting problems. It can take different forms, including escape, avoidance, procrastination and safety behaviours.[16] Escape might include the use of drugs and alcohol, and safety behaviours might involve superstitious behaviours (such as saying 'touch wood' when worried that something might not happen) or avoidance of people, places or activities that lead to anxious feelings. The basic purpose of avoidant behaviours is to make anxiety disappear, but it only works in the short term, and it causes more distress in the long term. For example, if the client is avoiding going to the local shops because this is where they had a panic episode, the anxiety can generalize to include other shopping centres, so there are more places to avoid.

Anxiety often triggers avoidance, and this is what can limit the client's life significantly and be disabling.

Exposure

In CBT, the key behavioural strategy of exposure is based on the concept that we become conditioned or have learnt to be afraid of certain triggers or situations, and our brains need to be reconditioned or rewired to not be fearful. The way this is done is through exposure, which involves activating the fear and habituating to it in a controlled way.[17] In other words, the best way to do 'exposure therapy' is gradually, using small steps.

Exposure therapy can occur in a number of different ways; for example, a counsellor might take the person through a number of role-plays. This can be useful in social anxiety, as it allows the person to rehearse or practise what they would say or do in the feared situation. Another technique is 'mental rehearsal', which involves taking the person gently through the feared situation in a state of relaxation or hypnosis. In doing so, the person experiences the situation in a more relaxed state and is conditioned to feel relaxed in the situation.[18]

LLCC TIP

With graded exposure, it is vital to ensure that the client has been taught a number of techniques beforehand to help them deal with anxiety symptoms, including breathing and relaxation techniques, and some cognitive strategies.

Let's consider a fear of spiders and a client called Jill, who hates spiders. Her fear is so great, that if there is a spider in her house she must leave and call a friend to remove it. You would want to ask Jill a number of questions such as, 'Are there particular types of spiders you are afraid of? Which colour/size of spider do you find more frightening?' The answers help determine what factors increase or decrease her fear (for example, black versus brown spiders, large versus small). Out of this discussion the counsellor, together with Jill, would generate a list of possible scenarios in relation to spiders, and rank them from least anxiety-provoking to most anxiety-provoking. See the left-hand column of Table 12 for the list of factors, and the middle column for the ranked degree of anxiety the scenario triggers. Use the following rating: 0 = no anxiety, 10 = the most anxiety Jill has ever experienced. The counsellor would then work with Jill to develop a series of graded exposure steps, and examples of these are shown in the right-hand column of the table. She might want to ultimately deal with the spider using insect spray, or might want to remove the spider from the house.

In the example, notice how there are a number of small steps in the graded exposure program for Jill, with the least difficult scenario tackled first, followed by the next difficult and then the next . . . until ultimately she is able to deal with a spider in her house. In this way the graded exposure program is achievable. Jill will notice that her anxiety will rise when she does each step, but it will then fall. Each step is repeated until it causes less anxiety (at least 50 per cent less) and then Jill will move on to the next. Sometimes there might be a setback and the client will need to return to a previous step and redo it, then move on to the next one. The program will take a good length of time to work through, maybe several months. Jill will need assistance from the therapist to source the jars with spiders in them. Remember that Jill does not need to be able to have a spider sitting on her, but she needs to be able to deal with one in her house. A blank copy of this program is included in the Appendix (see p. 296).

Table 12: Jill's graded exposure program

Factor/scenario	Anxiety (0–10)	Graded exposure steps
Small brown spider at a distance	5	1. Looking at pictures of small brown spiders
Small black spider at a distance	6	2. Looking at pictures of small black spiders
Large brown spider at a distance	7	3. Looking at pictures of large brown spiders
Large black spider at a distance	8	4. Looking at pictures of large black spiders
Small brown spider close up	9	5. Viewing dead spiders in glass containers at the museum from a distance
Small black spider close up	10	6. Viewing dead spiders in glass containers at the museum close up
Large brown spider close up	10	7. Viewing live spiders in glass containers at the museum from a distance
Large black spider close up	10	8. Viewing live spiders in glass containers at the museum close up (<1 minute)
		9. Viewing live spiders in glass containers at the museum close up (for several minutes)
		10. Holding a jar containing a small dead spider
		11. Holding a jar containing a large dead spider
		12. Holding a jar containing a small live spider
		13. Holding a jar containing a large live spider (<1 minute)
		14. Holding a jar containing a large live spider (several minutes)
		15. Spraying a spider with insect spray at home or removing from the premises

Exposure is also used in the management of agoraphobia and OCD. This is more complex and involves identifying the compulsive behaviours used to relieve the internal triggers, such as worrying thoughts or feelings. A program of challenging the behaviours and exposure to different situations through a hierarchy is used. To learn more about this, refer to the texts that focus on the treatment of anxiety disorders listed in 'Resources' at the end of the chapter, seek some supervision, or refer to an experienced colleague in this area.

COGNITIVE STRATEGIES AND CBT

In terms of CBT, helpful cognitive strategies in managing stress and anxiety include the following.

Identify the stressors

Identify the stressors, and see if there are some things that can be managed better. There will be some things beyond the client's control, for example, if there are work deadlines that cannot be changed. But in this example perhaps identifying what they *can* control in relation to managing the deadlines may be useful, such as scheduling to have at least a short lunch break each day, or going to bed earlier, or delegating some tasks.

Using the three-bucket metaphor

In anxiety, an underlying belief that can push the person around is 'I must be in control at all times'. This is not actually possible, and the three-bucket metaphor can help the client learn to distinguish between what is within their control and what is not:

- Explain to the client that there are three buckets in life, each with a lid. The first bucket represents everything to do with them — their dreams, goals, ideas and interests. The second bucket represents other people and everything to do with them. The third bucket represents the world we live in, the social codes we live by (laws, morals) and the environment.
- The client can lift the lid off the first bucket and take a look inside at any time; they can spend a lot of time dealing with everything in this bucket and influence it greatly. With the second bucket, to do with others, they can help or hinder others, and can influence this bucket to some degree, but a lesser degree. Sometimes they will need to put the lid on this bucket and put it aside for a while. With the third bucket, the client can run for politics or plant trees, but again, there will be limits to what they can do.
- The message is that there are some things outside of our control, and sometimes we need to focus on our own bucket and put the others aside for a while.

Problem-solving

Problem-solving is helpful when the anxious feelings and related negative thoughts are overwhelming. Problem-solving is sometimes seen as a facet of CBT but is also a therapy in its own right. It helps the client to think through a problem clearly, and to know where to start in dealing with it. Problem-solving involves sorting out what the problems are and looking at logical, practical ways of dealing with them. It involves a number of tasks, with the aim of deciding on the best possible solution for the problem. This may not be a total or perfect solution, but it will be a start and it will usually be helpful and make a difference.[19]

There are some general rules for problem-solving:

- Start with more straightforward problems rather than complex ones.
- Set aside time without distraction to work through problem-solving.
- Deal with problems one at a time, and go through each step one at a time.
- When making a list of possible solutions, write down all ideas even if some seem a bit wild! In the end an achievable solution needs to be chosen, but the process of writing down all possibilities often generates good ideas.
- When planning how to carry out the solution, it is important to be realistic — are the resources (time, money, etc.) available?
- Include plans for how to deal with difficulties or negative responses that might arise.
- Think about how positive outcomes will be managed, as these might involve adjusting to change.
- As with goal setting, it is useful to set a time by which to carry out the solution.
- Remember that even a partial success is a win, and the process of problem-solving is a learning process.[20]

The steps involved in problem-solving are as follows:

- Define the problem in everyday terms.
- Make a list of all possible solutions.
- Evaluate the solutions; that is, think about the advantages and disadvantages of each solution.
- Choose the best possible solution.
- Plan how to carry it out; this involves breaking the solution down into steps.
- Review progress.[21]

Managing negative thinking

We all have automatic thinking habits that can be unhelpful and which can lead us to worry more than is necessary. In anxiety, unhelpful thinking habits may include all-or-nothing thinking, mental filtering or catastrophizing. These can be driven by underlying beliefs such as 'All significant people in my life must love me and approve of me', 'I must always be competent and achieving in every area of my life', 'My life should progress easily and smoothly', 'It is better not to take risks' and 'I should always be in control'. In anxiety, the beliefs often relate to a sense of being threatened and lacking the ability to deal with threats; for example, 'I should always watch out if I am to avoid something awful happening' or 'If I feel anxious, this means I am losing control'.

The steps to deal with such thinking in CBT are as follows:

- Suggest the client become more aware of their thinking via keeping a thought diary several times a week, for example, and discuss the diary entries in counselling. The counsellor explains that thoughts are not facts, but actually assumptions, and that they are often automatic.

- Help the client develop an understanding of the types of unhelpful thinking patterns that can arise. Refer to page 51 and go through the table of thinking patterns with clients. If the client is using 'what if?' frequently, draw attention to worry about the future being helpful sometimes, but often being fruitless. It is important to focus on the present moment.

- Raise the client's awareness of the particular patterns they are susceptible to, and how these affect their levels of stress and anxiety. Also consider whether there are common situations in which they experience more unhelpful thinking, and what the triggers in these situations might be.

- Develop more helpful thinking by considering how accurate or helpful the thoughts are. The following questions can be useful:
  - 'What is the evidence for and against the thoughts?'
  - 'Ask yourself: Am I being too black and white, or am I labelling, mental filtering or catastrophizing?'
  - 'Is there another way to think about the situation?'
  - 'If a friend was saying this thought to you, what would you say to them?' This is a really helpful question for clients as they are likely to be more generous with friends than with themselves.

The aim is to reframe the unhelpful thoughts into more helpful thoughts. It is not about positive thinking all the time, but more balanced thinking, as negative thoughts sometimes give us useful information to take into account. More helpful thinking often emerges from the client having an expanded view of themselves or the situation they are in; for example, a mother with high expectations of herself might think 'I am no good at being a mother, I should be doing better'. When she understands the pressures on her from society, others and herself, she might be more balanced in her thinking, such as 'I am doing my best and it is a very hard job. Sometimes I feel overwhelmed by it, but that is okay. I am actually doing pretty well.'

An example of managing negative thinking follows, taken from Bill's story.

Note that the information in the first three columns come from the thought diary Bill kept for a few days prior to his most recent appointment. A copy of this pro forma to use with clients is provided in the Appendix (see p. 297).

Table 13: Managing Bill's negative thinking

Date/ time	What are you doing?	What are you thinking?	How do you feel?	Any unhelpful thinking patterns?	More helpful thoughts	How do you feel/ how are you now?
Sunday, 8 p.m.	Watching TV with the family	Ron (boss) will want my report first thing in the morning. I don't think it is good enough. What if he isn't happy? I could lose my job. I am over the whole thing, I don't want to go in.	Anxious, flat	Jumping to conclusions, black-and-white thinking, catastrophizing	I have work tomorrow; the report is done and I have done enough. Time to relax and enjoy Sunday night with my family.	Calmer, less worried.

Addressing the cascade of symptoms

In Panic Disorder there can be a cascade of anxiety symptoms, and cognitive and behavioural techniques can assist the client to manage this. The cascade involves having physical symptoms of the fight or flight response, triggering anxious thinking and feelings of anxiety. As the symptoms progress, the thinking becomes more catastrophic and the anxiety worsens.

Table 14: Cascade of symptoms, thoughts and feelings

Symptom	Thought	Feeling
Short of breath	'Oh no, it's back'.	Worried
Palpitations	'It's getting worse, it's my heart'.	Anxious
Chest discomfort	'What if I am having a heart attack?'	
Sweating		Terrified
Dizzy		

To interrupt the panic cascade and to prevent worsening of symptoms, follow these guidelines:

- Help the client become more aware of this process through psycho-education.

LLCC TIP

On a whiteboard write up the three headings, 'symptoms, thoughts and feelings', and then take the client through what happened in a recent panic episode. Ask the client to identify the first symptom, then the thought that occurred in response to this, and then the feeling. Work with the next symptom in a similar way, and keep going from left to right.

- Encourage the client to use the breathing techniques they have learnt to interrupt the cascade right at the start.
- Encourage the client to prepare a card with more helpful thoughts written on it to carry around with them (for example, in their wallet or handbag) and pull out at the onset of panic.

LLCC TIP

It can be helpful for the client to have a card with helpful thoughts written on it, such as 'Remember to use my breathing technique, I'm safe and okay, the feelings will pass very soon.'

The concept of '**surfing**' the anxious feelings is very helpful, and involves being aware of the feelings, observing them, catching them early, and staying just ahead of them as you would do if surfing a wave. In the case of anxiety you stay ahead of the feelings by using relaxation or cognitive techniques.

The client may also benefit from learning about **assertiveness training and communication skills** that can help them to deal with challenging situations more effectively, thereby reducing stress. There will be more on this in Chapter 6.

Mindfulness-based Cognitive Therapy

MBCT focuses on teaching the client to become more aware of thoughts (including ruminating thought patterns) and feelings, and to relate to them as 'mental events' which can be witnessed rather than as aspects of the self. It incorporates the practice of mindfulness and being with experience — that is, it encourages the individual to be aware of difficult thoughts and feelings, and to witness them in a different way and to foster a sense **self-compassion**.

Here is an example of a script for an MBCT technique that can be helpful for clients experiencing anxious feelings and thoughts.

Worry tends to involve a repetitive, circular thinking pattern, also known as rumination. We go around and around over the same thing with similar thoughts, not getting any further along. This is different from problem-solving with a practical outcome.

Let's label this circular type of thinking as 'just worrying'.

So when you are feeling anxious, observe your thoughts and if you notice that you are ruminating, label your thoughts as 'just worrying'. Then focus your attention on the breath, the breath in and the breath out, and relax with each breath out. Or you might like to change the subject of your thinking and focus on something else.

Apply this technique whenever you find yourself 'just worrying' and see how it helps you over the coming weeks.[22]

Solution-focused Therapy

Solution-focused Therapy, which is centred on solutions rather than the problem, can be helpful in stress and anxiety. Solution-focused Therapy:

- relies on identifying the issues, and then considers what the client will do about the issues and how they will carry out their plans
- involves looking at the client's resources, skills and strengths, and support networks
- involves asking coping questions, such as how the client has managed stress and anxiety in the past

■ focuses on how the client would like things to be different and what is required to make this happen.

Acceptance and Commitment Therapy

The ACT model was outlined in Chapter 3 (see p. 53). Its central aim is to develop more psychological flexibility and live a richer and more meaningful life. Key questions the counsellor asks during the assessment phase include, 'What valued direction do you want to move in?' and 'What is standing your way?' The first question relates to the client's values and the values-based goals which have been identified, while the second relates to the unhelpful thoughts the client is experiencing, the experiences they are trying to avoid (such as sensations or feelings), and the actions they are taking which may be unhelpful.[23]

ACT incorporates six key processes, and all can be helpful in anxiety:

1. Mindfulness, or contact with the present moment.
2. Defusion of feelings and thoughts.
3. Acceptance of uncomfortable feelings and thoughts, and the difficult things in life.
4. Self-as-context (the part of the mind that notices thoughts and feelings, that is calm and non-judgmental).
5. Values, or living a life consistent with what is important to the individual.
6. Committed action, as effort and action are central to change.[24]

The counsellor can begin by explaining each of these (further information follows). The counselling process will involve taking the client through a series of exercises to enable the client to experience the steps, and the focus will be on the client learning to apply them in their life.

VALUES

At the outset, the LLCC approach incorporates values into discussion about values-based goal-setting with the client. **Values** help us to have clear priorities in life as to how we allocate our time and energy.[25] To help the client identify their values, ask them to consider what have been the most rewarding parts of their life so far, what has brought them joy, what has inspired them or gives them meaning. Looking at Table 2 on page 33 can assist here, and there are other values exercises you may want to utilize (refer to *ACT Made Simple* by Russ Harris, 2009). The aim is to help the client to understand what they value the most in life, and that prioritizing these areas will help them feel less stressed because they are no longer trying to spread themselves too thin. Values are central and it is important for us to learn to regularly remind ourselves to come back to our values, especially when we feel lost or overwhelmed.

MINDFULNESS

By being mindful and engaging in the present, the client is less likely to worry about the past or the future.[26] In teaching mindfulness, begin by explaining the concept and its benefits (see p. 41). Counselling is a process of the client growing, and mindfulness is a key tool in learning new skills, such as cognitive skills. It has been suggested that the counsellor guides the client through a brief mindfulness skill at the start of each session, and in addition the counsellor might take the client through a number of mindfulness exercises as part of management.

LLCC TIP

Showing a YouTube video about mindfulness and the brain (such as 'Look what happens in your brain when you change your mind' by Dr Joe Dispenza (2009)) can be very powerful in explaining the benefits of mindfulness.

Teaching mindfulness skills is one of the keys to change, and these might include mindfulness in everyday life and mindfulness meditations. Mindfulness in everyday life could include eating and drinking in a mindful way (taking time and using the senses), spending mindful time with children or partner, or doing household or work tasks mindfully. There are many mindfulness meditations, and one has already been included with the breathing techniques discussed earlier. Here is another:

Make yourself comfortable and allow your eyes to close. Take a little while to become aware of the sensations in the body, and let yourself be still. Become aware of each part of the body and let go of any muscle tension, from the muscles in the face down through the shoulders and arms, the chest and abdomen, down through the legs to the feet and toes. Allow relaxation to flow through the body, letting any tension ease away. Be aware if your mind wanders away from your focus on muscle relaxation. That is okay and happens from time to time. Be patient with yourself and gently refocus your attention on letting go.

For a while, too, be aware of the breath. As you gently breathe in and out, feel the air warm as you breathe in through your nose, feel the air pass down through the lungs, using your tummy breathing, and then breathe out and let go, relax.

Now practise mindfulness of sounds. Bring your attention to your ears and your hearing. Listen to the sounds around you. Simply be open to sounds as they arise, and let them come into your awareness. Now release the awareness of sounds, and be aware of any thoughts that come into the mind; observe them and sit with them for a while. You can be aware of thoughts and you can allow them to move on, just as you would observe clouds floating across the sky and then disappearing into the distance.

Then, when you are ready to be alert, simply become aware of the body again and slowly open the eyes, feeling comfortable and in the here and now.

DEFUSION

Defusion is the opposite of 'fusion', which means being attached. The client can become 'fused' or very attached to their thoughts. A thought can seem to be the absolute truth when it is not necessarily. In ACT, defusion means separating or stepping back from thoughts, images and memories, and holding them gently rather than tightly. The metaphors of watching thoughts as if they were clouds floating across the sky, or a bus or going past, can be helpful. The client is asked to notice their thoughts. The counsellor uses questions such as, 'Can you notice what your thoughts are now?' or 'What is your mind telling you now?' The individual is also asked about whether the thought is helpful or, if the thought is followed, 'Will it take you in the direction of a rich and meaningful life, or will it keep you suffering?'[27]

ACCEPTANCE

Acceptance refers to making room for feelings, even the painful ones (such as anxiety), and reducing the struggle with them. This process also stems from the behavioural approach of exposure, highlighted earlier in this chapter. It is often a challenge as we want to avoid feeling uncomfortable, but it is by sitting with the discomfort that it can lessen. Acceptance can be assisted by mindfulness, defusion, and the next aspect of ACT: self-as-context.

SELF-AS-CONTEXT

Self-as-context relates to the mind and the concept that there are two separate parts to the human mind or human consciousness: the 'thinking self' or thinking mind, and the 'observing self'. Clients may know the thinking self well, due to having a constant stream of automatic thoughts. The observing self is the part of the mind which observes feelings, thoughts, sensations, memories, urges, sights, sounds, smells and tastes. This is the part that is able to 'step back' and observe these things and remain separate from them. This part does not get hooked up in what the thinking or judgmental mind is saying. The observing self enables self-awareness.[28]

TAKING ACTION

ACT also teaches the client that part of leading a rich life is taking action, and the action needs to be guided by their values. Harris says that it means 'doing what it takes', even if it brings up some discomfort.[29] Making an appointment with a counsellor and arriving at the appointment, reading self-help books, or doing some regular relaxation are examples of committed action. Values-based goal-setting can assist, and the behavioural strategies described earlier also fit with the process of committed action.[30] The client can also choose to take action in the present moment to decrease their stress levels, whereas we have less control over the past or the future.

ACT utilizes a number of metaphors to explain these processes. Examples include the following, as outlined below.

Hands as thoughts

Imagine that your hands are your thoughts. Cover your eyes with your hands for a moment. Then imagine what it would be like to go around all day with your hands over your eyes. How would it limit you? What would you miss out on? This is like fusion — we become so caught up in our thoughts that we lose contact with our here and now experiences, and we cannot act effectively. Then rest your hands on your lap, and notice the here and now. When you practise defusion, you can function fully.

Struggling in quicksand

Remember the old-fashioned movies where the bad guy falls into quicksand, and the more he struggles, the quicker he sinks? In quicksand the worst thing to do is struggle; but if you lie back, put your arms out and relax (a bit like acceptance), you remain afloat. It doesn't come naturally as your instinct is to struggle, but the aim is to quit the struggle and experience less suffering.

ACT AND ANXIETY

On the next page are some examples of ACT techniques that can be utilized with clients experiencing anxiety. It is important for the client to practise these with curiosity and mindfulness. Identify which of the above ACT processes are being incorporated into each, and when taking clients through them, discuss which particular ones they find most helpful.

Thought-noticing exercise

Make yourself comfortable and close your eyes. Imagine a recent experience that triggered some worrying thoughts (choose an uncomfortable, but not distressing, experience). Notice the thoughts. Identify one of them and add the prefix, 'I am having the thought that . . .'. Then identify another thought. This time, say the thought out loud in the voice of a cartoon or television character. Notice your response when you do this. Now think about the worrying situation again and identify another thought. This time, try singing the thought to a tune you know well, such as 'Happy Birthday'.

When you have finished exploring these ideas, focus on the sounds you can hear around you, open your eyes and bring your attention back to the room.[31]

'Add thoughts to leaves' exercise

Make yourself comfortable and let your eyes close. Imagine you are sitting beside a gentle stream, and there are leaves flowing past on the surface of the water. Over the next few minutes, observe each thought that comes into your mind. Then take a thought and imagine placing it on a leaf, and let it float by. If a feeling pops up, observe the feeling and say, 'Here's a feeling of . . .' and place it on a leaf. When you are ready, gently open your eyes and bring your attention back to the room.[32]

'Being with an emotion' exercise

Identify the feeling you want to work with, such as anxiety. Notice the feeling and where you feel it in the body. You might feel it in the chest or stomach. What shape or colour does it look like? Now imagine gently breathing into it, and keep breathing in and out to that spot in the body. Then allow some space around the feeling and sit with it for a while. Just allow it to be there, and breathe. Notice what happens with the feeling. When you are ready, open your eyes and bring your attention back to the room.[33]

 LLCC TIP

The 'Being with an emotion' exercise is one of the most useful and powerful techniques I have come across in my entire career. It can be applied in a range of situations and emotions.

'Thoughts and rooms' exercise

Imagine your mind is a white room with a door at either end of the room. Thoughts come IN through one door and go OUT the other door. Watch each thought as it enters the IN door. As you pay attention to the thought, label it as either a judgmental or a non-judgmental thought. Observe the thought as it makes its way across the room to the OUT door and leaves. Don't judge the judgment, don't analyze it or hold on to it. Don't believe or disbelieve it; just notice the thought and acknowledge it. It's just a moment in time, a brief visitor in the white room that is your mind. It is nearly impossible to stop your mind coming up with these judgments; it will constantly evaluate and judge your experiences. Notice if you are judging yourself for having the thought. Don't try to change the judgment, justify it or argue with it. Just acknowledge it for what it is and label it: there is 'judging', there is 'worry'.

Recognizing judgmental thoughts and not getting trapped or hooked in by them is the goal of this exercise. The length of time each thought stays in the room and the intensity of your emotional reaction will guide you as to whether you are getting hooked by certain thoughts. Continue noticing, continue the deep breathing and continue labelling. A thought is just a thought; it is not a fact or the truth. It is not the truth about you; it does not totalize you as a person and it is not the boss of you. Each thought does not mean you have to react. Observe your thoughts as if they were visitors passing in and out of the white room. Let them have their brief moment of your attention; they are fine the way they are. Let the judging thoughts and all the other uninvited visitors just be; let them enter the room and leave the room without reaction, without struggle. Then you are ready to greet and label the next thought . . . and the next. Keep doing this exercise until you feel a real emotional shift and a growing distance from your thoughts. Continue doing the exercise until the judgments are no longer bossing, no longer demanding action and no longer important. Wait until the thoughts and judgments are fleeting and take but a moment for you to watch them come in and out of the room. When you are ready, gently open your eyes and come back to the here and now.[34]

The struggle switch

Imagine that at the back of your mind is a 'struggle switch'. When it is on, you are going to struggle against any emotional distress that comes your way. Anxiety may show up, and with the struggle switch on, you will do the best to get rid of it. But suppose the switch is off and anxiety shows up; you might say 'Okay, there's a knot in my stomach, my mind is telling me scary stories, it's unpleasant, but I'm not going to waste energy struggling with it. Instead I am going to take action and do something meaningful.' So with the struggle switch off, our anxiety might come and go, but we do not create additional suffering for ourselves.[35]

Worry smog

In his book *The Confidence Gap*, Harris describes what he calls the 'worry smog'. This is like a thick cloud of thoughts that prevents us from thinking clearly. To clear the worry smog, follow these steps:

Step 1: Be clear about what 'worrying' is. Worrying means fusing with thoughts of bad things that might happen. It is not just the thoughts.

Step 2: Identify the costs of worrying; that is, what we miss out on from not being present, such as wasted time or disrupted sleep.

Step 3: Unhook from the reasons to worry. For example, if worrying is viewed as helpful for preparing for the worst, it will be much more effective to move from worrying to active planning or constructive problem-solving.

Step 4: Distinguish worrying from taking care; for example, worrying about your health versus taking care of your health through healthy nutrition and exercise.

Step 5: Defuse from worrying itself; that is, notice worrying and name it.[36]

Interpersonal Therapy

IPT has been shown to be useful in the management of anxiety disorders, in particular Panic Disorder, SAD and PTSD. If the formulation highlights relationships as contributing to the stress and anxiety, it is very helpful to explore IPT, which focuses on improving interpersonal relationships to relieve symptoms. It categorizes the relationship difficulties into four potential types:

- grief due to loss
- interpersonal disputes or conflicts
- role transitions, such as becoming a mother or father, or changing jobs
- interpersonal sensitivities, such as deficiencies in social skills or networks.

Reflection on Bill's story

Bill had experienced role transitions with a new job and having a family. There was loss and grief related to his father, and some interpersonal conflicts were beginning to arise with his wife. As you read the next section, consider how IPT might assist Bill.

Two tools are used in the initial stages of IPT to help gather information and contribute to the formulation. These not only gather very useful information but can also assist understanding and insight — just be aware that they can be confronting. (An interpersonal inventory template is provided in the Appendix; see p. 298)

1. The **interpersonal inventory**:
   - provides a review of important current and past relationships
   - uncovers frequency of contact, shared activities, expectations (fulfilled or not)
   - examines satisfactory or unsatisfactory aspects of relationships
   - brings to light ways the client would like the relationship/s to change
   - works to identify relationship between the anxiety and the interpersonal issues.
2. A **timeline** provides a visual representation of the links between life events, relationships and the anxiety. It differs from other timelines in that relationships are included. (A sample timeline is provided on p. 178)

The counsellor and client together identify which of the problem areas are relevant. Management involves psycho-education, and strategies to manage the problem areas.

- Any loss and grief is addressed using techniques such as those described in Chapter 10.
- Interpersonal disputes are explored and the client assisted with modifying any unhelpful expectations in the relationship or communication issues. More information on this is provided in Chapter 12.
- Role transitions are discussed and dealing with these may involve managing grief, or acceptance of loss of the old role. It may also involve assisting the client to consider new roles more positively, to explore related feelings and enhance low self-belief (see Chapter 13).
- Addressing interpersonal sensitivities might involve raising awareness of challenges in social situations and learning new social skills, or reducing social isolation.

In addressing these areas, IPT incorporates range of techniques. These include:

- exploration of the patient's perceptions and expectations of others (through the inventory and discussion)
- encouragement of affect; that is, feelings are explored and expressed
- clarification of issues and identification of problems in relationships
- problem-solving (covered earlier in this chapter)
- communication analysis, which aims to identify whether the client's current problems are related to their ability to communicate. It looks out for incorrect assumptions, indirect verbal communication, unhelpful silence/shutting down behaviours; the counsellor asks the client about

their communication patterns, helps them to understand the effect of their communication and works with them to establish more productive patterns

■ behaviour change techniques, including role-play, which provides an opportunity for the client and therapist to act out interactions and to examine and address the patient's communication style and explore effective interactions.

Narrative Therapy

Narrative therapy provides many useful perspectives in managing stress and anxiety.

Deconstruction of the **dominant story** (that of stress or anxiety) and reconstruction of an **alternative story** is powerful. For example, you might find that a client with anxiety is also someone who has strengths of sensitivity and creativity. Finding the alternative story might also involve deconstructing the 'truths' the person has adopted that influence their story, and exploring the influences of the problem in the person's life and relationships. It may involve identifying some of the negative conclusions the client might have reached about their identity, under the influence of the problem, such as 'having anxiety means I am weak', and more broadly redeveloping their strengths and resources.[37]

Deconstruction of the dominant story related to the anxiety, and reconstruction of an alternative story, is powerful. This often incorporates the client's strengths and resources.

Narrative therapy can inform the client's understanding about how various influences in society can impact their thinking and beliefs about themselves. If the influences are imagined as an umbrella above the individual, then that 'umbrella of life' includes school, family and friends, government, religion, culture and media. There are dominant views about the role of women and men in society, for example, or what constitutes success. If a client measures themselves against these notions, and does not think they are measuring up well, this can contribute to feelings of stress or anxiety (or depression).

LLCC TIP
Use a whiteboard or paper to draw an umbrella with a two people standing under it. Then take the client through an exercise about how society views the 'ideal woman' and the 'ideal man'. This will highlight how we are influenced by society's views, such as: the ideal woman is slim, pretty, capable, a good mother . . . the ideal man is strong, muscular, successful . . . Discuss how these ideas have arisen.

The language the counsellor uses to talk about stress and anxiety is important. **Externalizing language**, such as discussing how 'the anxiety' is pushing them around or impacting the person's life, helps to place the anxiety outside of the individual, implying they are not the same as the anxiety. Externalizing the problem or placing it outside the client is particularly important when the experience of the problem is totalizing the person's life. An example is talking about what the anxiety might look like if it was sitting outside the client on the floor, or giving it a name.

Mapping the effects of the stress or anxiety in the client's life and relationships is helpful. For example, a client with anxiety might map out and consider the consequences of the problem on their relationships. This might look similar to the IPT timeline.

Metaphors, such as walking out on the anxiety, freeing life from it or taming it, can be used.

Reconstruction of an alternative story to the one dominated by anxiety may involve **re-authoring** conversations that will help the client to discover unique outcomes which would not have been predicted under the influence of the anxiety. For example, despite being pushed around by anxiety, the client might have nonetheless become a competent tennis player or musician, or decide to help others with their own struggles. Look for exceptions to the dominant story, as there are always some. Questions might explore times when (the problem) was not a problem for them, and what that was like.[38]

Much of the Narrative Therapy process involves therapeutic conversations, and being curious and using questioning. Here are some examples to use in stress and anxiety.

- 'What is the impact of stress or anxiety on your life?'
- 'How has stress or anxiety impacted on your view of yourself?'
- 'If stress or anxiety were to continue to dominate your life, how would this influence your future experience of yourself?'

- 'Think of a time when in some small way you have been able to stand up to the stress or anxiety and have stopped it pushing you around.
  - What qualities, skills or abilities did it take for you to resist stress or anxiety in this way?
  - How can you use these qualities, skills, abilities or strategies in the future to continue to challenge stress or anxiety?'
- 'Stress or anxiety can dominate our lives and make it hard for us to see how we have resisted its tricks and traps. Think back through your life to other times when you were able to outsmart stress or anxiety, and describe what happened. If you were to continue to challenge stress or anxiety in this way, how would your life be different?'
- 'Think of someone who is special to you and knows you well. What would they predict for your life if they were made aware of your success over stress or anxiety?'
- 'What kind of person are you in the process of becoming, and what would your special person/s say about this?'
- 'How are you going to "catch up" the significant people in your life about your new story? What events will you tell them about so that they can appreciate you are no longer being tricked and trapped by stress or anxiety?'
- 'How are you going to celebrate your achievements? Are you going to have some kind of ritual or ceremony, and who are the important people you will invite to be an audience to your new story?'[39]

Positive Therapy

Positive Therapy can be helpful in stress and anxiety. It can help identify strengths and encourage greater use of them, as people who use their strengths experience less stress.[40]

LLCC TIP

A strengths questionnaire can assist (see www. authentichappines.sas.upenn.edu), or try strengths cards — put them on the desk or floor and ask the client to pick out which ones they relate to. There are also strengths phone apps (see 'Resources' at the end of this chapter).

Once identified, a useful exercise is to ask the client to consider three ways they can use each of their top few strengths.

Positive Therapy fosters positive emotions such as those gained through savouring enjoyable moments, and practising gratitude and kindness. Even when life is very stressful, it is still possible to be grateful for even the smallest things — the sunshine or a friendly word from someone. Gratitude helps people to cope with stress and trauma; appreciating life can be used as a coping method to help positively reinterpret negative life events.[41] Encourage the client to write down or share out loud three things they are grateful for regularly; the optimum frequency to write in a gratitude journal once a week.[42] Also, encourage the client to practise kindness regularly. Lyubomirsky developed an exercise called the 'five acts of kindness' which encourages performing five acts of kindness each day, such as donating blood, helping a neighbour or helping a friend.

LLCC TIP
Suggest that the client keeps a gratitude diary, regularly recording three things they are grateful for. Encourage them to choose a beautiful notebook to write in to help make it special.

Leisure and creativity, which can relax and engage us, are encouraged in Positive Therapy. Examples of exercises related to leisure and creativity include cooking, writing, singing, colouring, gardening, or playing a musical instrument you enjoy.

LLCC TIP
Try the 'observing the rose' exercise devised by psychotherapist, Stephanie Dowrick. Go for a walk and collect a flower. Take it home, then place it in front of you and describe it as someone who has never seen or smelt a flower like it. This helps engage the client to focus on the present moment, requiring that they take a fresh look at something they are already familiar with and therefore often overlook. It takes creativity to do this, too! [43]

Other aspects of Positive Therapy include the following:

- Mindfulness, self-care and positive coping skills, such as meditation or problem-solving, are emphasized.
- There is a focus on the role of values and **authenticity**, which describes being true to oneself by understanding our interior, psychological life and presenting our true self to others. With authenticity comes the pursuit of goals that are more meaningful and more integrated with the self; the result is greater wellbeing.[44]
- **Resilience**, which refers to the capacity to maintain competent function despite major life stressors, is fostered.[45] The metaphor of a bridge is helpful, in which stressors create a load on the bridge and the pillars of the bridge (the client's internal and external resources) give it strength. When faced with threats, those individuals with more resilient personality styles worry less and rebound faster (they 'bounce back'). Developing resilience is key in **prevention** of distress and mental health issues. Resilient people are characterized by:
    - being highly attuned to ever-changing circumstances and being flexible
    - reacting to what is happening 'in the now'
    - adopting a 'wait and see' attitude
    - having helpful coping mechanisms
    - focusing on the reality of the present moment
    - reframing bad events as opportunities
    - making use of both positivity and openness.[46]

Fortunately individuals can become more resilient through experiencing more positive emotions and welcoming positivity, even when the worst is feared. Connecting with others, developing good problem-solving skills and practising acceptance can assist.[47]

Hypnotherapy

Hypnotherapy is helpful in stress and anxiety. Consider using hypnotherapy in the following ways:

- To teach the person **relaxation** techniques. The deepening in hypnosis often utilizes progressive muscle relaxation, breathing and visualization techniques, such as those described earlier in this chapter.
- The client is taught **self-hypnosis** to use on a regular basis (see p. 78).
- Direct suggestions can be given about feeling more calm, relaxed and confident each day or in certain situations.
- **Indirect suggestions** or metaphors can be used. For example, a client

with Generalized Anxiety Disorder could be involved in a metaphor about going on a journey and coming across different challenging situations, and finding creative ways to deal with them in a calm and relaxed way.

■ A post-hypnotic suggestion (or **anchor**) might also be used to suggest relaxation and success. When the client is in the hypnotic state, and feeling relaxed and safe, such as in a special place in nature, they are instructed to gently squeeze together the thumb and index finger of the right hand to bring a wave of calmness and confidence, in or out of the relaxed state.

■ When there are specific anxiety disorders, such as SAD or specific phobias, hypnosis can integrate strategies from **CBT** or **ACT** such as:

— Exposure, which is done in the same graded way as outlined previously (see p. 93). Exposure can initially be done in a gentle and dissociated way, by asking the client to imagine a movie screen to which they have the controls, and they can watch a film of the feared situation while in the relaxed state. They can watch it forwards and even backwards.

— If there is performance anxiety, for example, the client can practise a talk or performance in the imagination while in the relaxed state. Prior to using this technique, ensure the details of the scenario are correct — where will they be, what does it look like, who is there, what will they play, and so on. Take them through the scenario and utilize strategies to aid relaxation, such as breathing, helpful thinking and using their 'anchor'.

— The steps involved in problem-solving could be reinforced through suggestions, if appropriate, and an example from the client's life used. Suggestions can also be given, for example, about becoming totally involved in the talk or music and being in the flow with it.

— The CBT model can be explained in hypnosis and the concepts reinforced, such as that thoughts are not facts.

— Having taken the client through unhelpful thinking styles out of hypnosis, and knowing what styles tend to be traps for that person, the counsellor can give suggestions in hypnosis about how those styles can develop and the troubles they can lead to. This can be followed by suggestions about being more aware of them in everyday life, and learning to outsmart or soften them by thinking differently.

— Ways to challenge unhelpful thoughts can be reinforced, along with more helpful ways of thinking.

— In Panic Disorder, suggestions can be given about the client carrying a toolkit of strategies such as breathing techniques and more helpful thinking, and pulling the tools out whenever needed.

— The various ACT scripts which teach mindfulness, defusion, acceptance and self-as-context can be woven into hypnotherapy. In fact, these techniques are very hypnotic.

■ Work can be done around self-belief in hypnotherapy, through direct suggestion and metaphor (see Chapter 13).

Bibliotherapy and e-mental health

Bibliotherapy and e-mental health are very useful in stress and anxiety. Within and between sessions I often utilize the following books: *Release Your Worries* (Howell and Murphy, 2011), *The Happiness Trap Pocketbook* (Harris and Aisbett, 2013) and *Living With It* (Aisbett, 1993). A suggestion is to talk about different chapters in the books, and then ask the client to read parts of them and do any exercises. These can then be discussed in the next session.

There are some excellent websites for psycho-education and also for therapy, in particular CBT. The websites for the Centre for Clinical Interventions (CCI) and the Clinical Research Unit for Anxiety and Depression (CRUFAD) at Sydney's St Vincent's Hospital are both very good (see 'Resources' p. 118). Go through some of the CCI modules on anxiety with clients in sessions, or they might want to engage in the online programs such as those provided by CRUFAD.

In summary

Stress and anxiety are part of life, and can be troublesome for many clients. There are many strategies that can assist, and you will find that different clients will find different ones helpful. Let's reflect on Bill's story again, and see how the LLCC approach was able to help him.

Reflection on Bill's story

Bill was experiencing stress and generalized worry, and the more recent panic attacks triggered him to seek help. He found these frightening and feared he might die. There had been a lot of stress and change in the past two years, and he was self-medicating with alcohol in an effort both to sleep and to reduce his anxiety symptoms.

The counsellor began by exploring his story and identifying the key issues with him. The panic attacks were his main concern, so education about these was helpful to alleviate fear, along with discussion about his family history. He was taught some breathing and cognitive strategies to manage the panic episodes, and he found having these tools very helpful.

Bill and the counsellor met again to focus on mindfulness and relaxation strategies to put into practice each day. They also talked about the sleep issues and alcohol. Bill thought that if he started some exercise again it might relieve each of these issues. Further sessions focused on the cognitive aspects of CBT. Bill gradually improved.

LLCC TIPS: MANAGING STRESS AND ANXIETY

- Do more relaxing activities such as meditation, exercise or hobbies.
- Aim for a healthy lifestyle.
- Focus on doing things you value.
- Practise mindfulness.
- Connect with family and friends.
- Challenge negative thoughts.
- Use humour to de-stress.
- Prioritize and look after yourself.
- Learn to be assertive and to say 'no'.
- Practise self-compassion.

Resources

Books

Aisbett, B. 1993, *Living With It: A survivor's guide to panic attacks*, Angus and Robertson, Sydney, New South Wales.

Andrews, G., Lampe, L. et al. 2002, *The Treatment of Anxiety Disorders: Clinician's guides and patient manuals* (2nd ed.), Cambridge University Press, UK.

Edelman, S. 2013, *Change Your Thinking: Positive and practical ways to overcome stress, negative emotions and self-defeating behaviour using CBT*, HarperCollins Publishers, Sydney.

Eifert, G. and Forsyth, J. 2005, *Acceptance and Commitment Therapy for Anxiety Disorders: A practitioner's treatment guide to using mindfulness, acceptance and values-based behaviour change strategies*, New Harbinger Publications, California.

Harris, R. 2007, *The Happiness Trap: Stop struggling, start living*, Exisle Publishing, New South Wales.

Harris, R. 2009, *ACT Made Simple: An easy-to-read primer on Acceptance and Commitment Therapy*, New Harbinger Publications, California.

Harris, R. Aisbett, B. 2013, *The Happiness Trap Pocketbook*, Exisle Publishing, New South Wales.

Howell, C. 2009, *Keeping the Blues Away: The ten-step guide to reducing the relapse of depression*, Radcliffe, London.

Howell, C. 2014, *Meditation and Mindfulness: What's all the fuss about?* e-book available at www.drcatehowell.com.au

Howell, C. and Murphy, M. 2011, *Release Your Worries: A guide to letting go of stress and anxiety*, Exisle Publishing, New South Wales.

Lampe, L. 2008, *Take Control of Your Worry: Managing Generalised Anxiety Disorder*, Simon & Schuster, Sydney.

McKenzie, S. and Hassed, C. 2012, *Mindfulness for Life*, Exisle Publishing, New South Wales.

Wells, A. 1997, *Cognitive Therapy of Anxiety Disorders: A practice manual and conceptual guide*, John Wiley & Sons, West Sussex.

Websites

ACT and mindfulness: www.actmindfully.com.au

Australian Government Department of Veterans' Affairs, PTSD Coach: http://at-ease.dva.gov.au/veterans/resources/mobile-apps/ptsd-coach/

Australian Indigenous Mental Health: www.indigenous.ranzcp.org/index.php

Beyondblue: www.beyondblue.org.au

Blogs and mental health information: www.drcatehowell.com.au

Centre for Clinical Interventions, with excellent resources for clinicians and consumers on anxiety and CBT-based treatment: www.cci.health.wa.gov.au

Clinical Research Unit for Anxiety and Depression (University of NSW): https://crufad.org/

National Institute for Health and Care Excellence (NICE) guidelines on Anxiety Disorders: http://www.nice.org.uk/Guidance/qs53

New Zealand mental health resources: www.mentalhealth.org.nz/get-help/a-z

Self-help website UK (many resources on CBT): www.Getselfhelp.co.uk

South African Depression and Anxiety Group: www.sadag.org/

UK NHS website for general information: www.nhs.uk/Conditions/stress-anxiety-depression/Pages/low-mood-stress-anxiety.aspx

University of Pennsylvania, strengths questionnaire: www.authentichappiness.sas.upenn.edu

US Department of Defense, National Center for Telehealth & Technology: http://t2health.dcoe.mil/

Phone apps

Breathing Zone: www.breathing-zone.com

Meditation Oasis: www.meditationoasis.com/apps/

Take a Break meditations

iSleep Easy meditations for sleep

Smiling Mind: www.smilingmind.com.au

Breathe2Relax portable stress management tool: http://t2health.dcoe.mil/apps/breathe2relax

Black Dog Institute: www.blackdoginstitute.org.au/public/research/ehealth.cfm

Psych Central top ten mental health apps: http://psychcentral.com/blog/archives/2013/01/16/top-10-mental-health-apps/

Optimism apps: www.findingoptimism.com

Chapter 6
Overcoming depression

If you are depressed you are living in the past.
If you are anxious you are living in the future.
If you are at peace you are living in the present.

—LAO TZU

We experience various emotions, and some are perceived 'negative' emotions, such as sadness and depression, anger, guilt and shame. We often group emotions into 'good' and 'bad', but all emotions are valuable as they are part of life and give us information. Our emotions are not always set at 'happy', and life events can trigger sadness or depression. In the event of depressed mood, thorough assessment is vital to identify whether it has been triggered by recent events or is due to an underlying depressive illness.

Taylor's story

Twenty-two-year-old Taylor is studying and working in a health-related area. Her family lives a few hours away, and she is sharing accommodation with a housemate. Taylor is a very good athlete, and trains and competes regularly. She attends for assistance because she is feeling teary, not sleeping well, and struggling with motivation with her studies and sport.

The counsellor meets with Taylor and hears her story. A thorough assessment is carried out over the first couple of sessions, including the DASS, and the counsellor becomes concerned that Taylor has significant depression symptoms. The counsellor suggests that Taylor also see her GP for further assessment, including some blood tests and potentially medication.

The counsellor continues to meet with Taylor and together they identify some key issues to focus to focus on in their sessions, including the stress of studying and training, poor sleep, low motivation and social isolation.

Background

Henry Wadsworth Longfellow wrote:

> Be still, sad heart! and cease repining
> Behind the clouds is the sun still shining
> Thy fate is the common fate of all,
> Into each life some rain must fall.

Sadness is commonly experienced in life, often triggered by upsetting life events. It is important to differentiate this from persistent feelings of **depression**, which may or may not have precipitating events, and which can cause significant health issues. Feelings of sadness or brief depressive feelings are part of life, but when depressed mood persists for a period of time and is impacting a person's life and functioning, it is considered an illness.

The hallmarks of **Major Depressive Disorder** are persistent low mood and/or loss of enjoyment in activities a person usually enjoys, along with a range of other issues, such as sleep disturbance, low energy, poor concentration or feelings of hopelessness. Thoughts of self-harm or suicide can develop as a result.

Some people can have a genetic tendency to depression, which leads to greater vulnerability to it. Depression certainly feels awful, but there are many approaches and strategies that can assist, and mostly it will pass in weeks or months.

> # Depression involves persistently low mood and/or loss of enjoyment in activities usually enjoyed.

There are many myths about depression and these play a part in stigma in the community; for example, depression means 'weakness'. In fact, many people will experience depression, and having depression means the person is facing challenges that take courage to overcome. Actively managing depression can reduce its length. About 40 per cent of people will recover and not experience another episode; about 40 per cent will have a second episode of depression; and about 20 per cent will have a more chronic course.[1]

There are a number of life circumstances which put a person at greater risk of developing depression. Post childbirth is a time of vulnerability for depression, in both mothers and fathers. They experience fatigue and change, and both of these are stressful. Severe or chronic illness (for example, heart disease and cancer) and the associated challenges are also associated with depression. Loss and grief plays a significant part, too.

Those with depression are at risk of anxiety, substance use issues (such as overuse of alcohol, often to self-treat the symptoms) or problems such as gambling. This is also why it is important to intervene early. Anxiety can certainly trigger depression, so again intervening early with anxiety to prevent depression is vital. Examples include someone with Social Anxiety or Obsessive Compulsive Disorder becoming depressed by the impact of the anxiety on their life. Depression itself can be associated with agitated or anxious feelings.

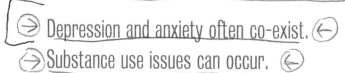

> # Depression and anxiety often co-exist. <
> # Substance use issues can occur. <

The symptoms of depression can be summarized as follows.
- **Affective** (emotions) — depression, anxiety, guilt, anger, hostility, irritability, inability to experience pleasure.
- **Behavioural** — agitation, facial expression, slowing down of movements,

speech and thought, crying.

- **Attitudes** towards self and world — self-criticism, low self-belief, feelings of helplessness, hopelessness, pessimism, thoughts of death or suicide.
- **Cognitive** — impaired thinking and concentration.
- **Bodily complaints** — loss of appetite, sleep disturbance, low energy or libido.[2]

LLCC management

There are some key areas to address with clients who are feeling depressed.

- **Support and reassurance.** Clients often report that central to their recovery is the sense that someone understands their distress, is supporting them and travelling with them. Reassurance that there is hope or light at the end of the tunnel is also very important.
- **Psycho-education.** Having good information is important, as understanding gives a greater sense of self-empowerment and can relieve associated anxiety. Providing information (such as that given previously) about depression is helpful, and there are numerous books or websites which can assist (see 'Resources' at the end of the chapter).
- **Addressing lifestyle.** A number of lifestyle interventions have been shown to help in depression.[3] Whatever the cause of depression, the depression itself tends to indicate that some changes in lifestyle are needed, and these might involve eating more nutritious food (despite not having an appetite) or reducing comfort eating of unhealthy foods.[4] Exercise is known to have a positive effect on mood, and so this can be encouraged.[5] Getting out into nature has also been shown to lift our spirits, and the client might want to combine this with exercise. It is also important to minimize the use of caffeine, alcohol, cigarettes and other drugs.
- **Sleep** is often disturbed in depression, so measures to regulate sleep are valuable (see p. 71). In addition, going for a walk in the morning light triggers melatonin production in the brain, which aids night-time sleep. Activities that reduce stress, such as those the client generally enjoys, or mindfulness and meditation, can be encouraged.
- Guiding the client in setting some basic **short-term goals** based on their values is helpful, such as spending time with a family member or walking the dog. It is important to encourage action. A client might think that because they don't feel like doing something, they cannot do it. But this is not actually true. How often do we do things we really don't feel like doing, such as cleaning or paying bills? Start with small steps and gradually build on them, and then the feeling of success may well reinforce more activity.

A range of psychological therapies can assist in depression, and we will explore **SFT, CBT, MBCT, ACT, IPT, Narrative Therapy, Hypnotherapy, Bibliotherapy** and **e-mental health.** Undertaking such therapies can help the person recover from depression and also contribute to them staying well in the future. To begin with, it can be helpful to keep a mood diary.[6] The client is asked to record their mood each day for a week. They rate their mood from 0 to 10, where 0 refers to no depression and 10 to the most severe depression, and record a rating twice each day. They can use the same diary to comment on sleep length and quality, and any significant events or activities of the day. A sample of Taylor's diary is provided below and a pro forma is in the Appendix (see p. 299).

Table 15: Taylor's mood diary

	Day 1	Day 2	Day 3	Day 4	Day 5	Day 6	Day 7
Mood (morning)	6/10	5/10	6/10	5/10	6/10	6/10	5/10
Mood (evening) (0-10)	6/10	5/10	7/10	4/10	7/10	5/10	4/10
Sleep	Could not sleep until 1 a.m.	Fell asleep 11 p.m., up at 5 a.m.	Asleep at midnight, up at 5 a.m.	1 a.m.– 6 a.m.	Midnight –7 a.m.	11 p.m. –8 a.m.	Midnight– 7 a.m.
Other (e.g. events, activities)	Doing study at home, worried about uni on Monday	Uni went okay, training after uni	Tired but could not sleep, then up early. Went for a run.	Felt very flat, upset with friend at uni, just tired.	More sleep, yay, uni better, training, then shopping	Study, cycling, out to dinner with friends, better sleep	Work, study, watched movie at home

As time passes the counsellor and client might see patterns, and hopefully improvement. Alternatively, mood can be mapped on a graph (refer to Appendix, p. 300) to provide a visual record. It can be helpful to use these records to give feedback to the client about progress. Consider also regularly using a monitoring assessment tool, such as the DASS, to record progress and to provide feedback (see p. 286).

LLCC TIP
It is helpful to monitor recovery regularly with an appropriate assessment tool, such as the DASS. It also provides feedback to the client about their progress.

Solution-focused Therapy

Aspects of SFT, which is focused on solutions, can be helpful. The key is identifying the issues, and then considering what the client will do about the issues and how they will carry out their plans. It involves looking at the client's resources and strengths, and making use of support networks. Coping skills are highlighted, and the **miracle question** can be helpful at times: 'Imagine that while you're sleeping a miracle happens: the problem you brought here has been solved. But because you are sleeping, you don't know that this has happened. So when you wake up, what would be different to tell you that a miracle has happened and your problem is solved?'[7]

Pam's story

Pam, 75, was feeling depressed. She had health problems, family and financial issues. She and her husband had lost money on investments. Discussion with the counsellor seemed to go around in circles, and they decided to use the miracle question. Pam answered: 'The house would be sold, the mortgage cleared, and we would own a smaller house.' Questions followed exploring what it meant to Pam that they were in their current financial position, and she replied: 'It means I am a failure.' A shift in the discussion followed, as the distress around this could be expressed and explored.

Cognitive Behaviour Therapy

There is a great deal of evidence for the benefits of CBT in managing depression.[8] In terms of behavioural interventions, a starting point is often encouraging the client to engage in a range of activities, including pleasurable ones. Activity or occupation is central to life, as our daily routine, our work and leisure time involve activities. They can give us a great sense of satisfaction and achievement, and pleasure. Loss of motivation and lethargy are common in depression. This means the individual with depression is less likely to do the activities that usually provide them with pleasure. A vicious cycle can result — the less active the individual becomes, the more depressed they feel and the less they do.[9]

It is important for the client to not only recognize the importance and benefits of activity, but to also give themselves permission to enjoy a range of activities, including relaxing, creative or pampering activities. People's lives can be greatly changed and their mood lifted through activity. The key is finding activities that are meaningful to the person — perhaps something creative, or doing something to help another person, or teaching a skill. The story below demonstrates the value of activity in depression.

Alfred's story

When working at a major city hospital many years ago as an OT, I was asked to see an elderly gentleman called Alfred from central Australia. He had had a heart attack and was struggling with mood post heart attack. As I spoke with him, I discovered that he was descended from Afghan camel traders, and as a young boy had learnt to create leather whips and saddles for the camels. Now he was elderly and feeling depressed after a heart attack.

At the same time I was asked to see two young men in the hospital's burns unit, both of whom had burns to their arms. I chose to get the three men together, and I asked Alfred to help by teaching the young men some leather work, as this activity would assist function to return to their upper limbs. Alfred obliged over several weeks, and the change in both him and the young men was remarkable. Alfred was doing something of value, while also tapping into his creative skills again. The depression lifted and he returned home after his cardiac rehabilitation.

ACTIVITY SCHEDULING

There are some guidelines for planning daily activities, or 'activity scheduling'.
- Don't plan for the whole week at once; just plan for a single day at a time.
- Plan the activities a day ahead.

- Plan them in one-hour time slots.
- Schedule some activities that give pleasure.
- Start with easy-to-achieve activities, and gradually include more difficult tasks.
- Don't worry if an activity is missed; the client can still continue with other scheduled activities.
- Note any extra activities that were done during the day.
- Work towards getting back to a more normal routine.
- Try activity scheduling for at least a week.

An activity scheduling chart is provided below in Table 16. Note that the pleasure rating refers to the degree of pleasure associated with doing the activity; use a scale of 0 to 5, with 0 for no pleasure and 5 for maximum pleasure. The achievement rating refers to the sense of achievement gained from doing the activity; again, this is rated from 0 to 5, with 0 for no achievement and 5 for maximum achievement.

Table 16: Activity schedule[10]

Date/time	Planned activity/ies	Tick when done, or note other activities	Rate pleasure and sense of achievement (0–5 for each)
7–8 a.m.			
8–9 a.m.			
9–10 a.m.			
10–11 a.m.			
11 a.m.–12 p.m.			
12–1 p.m.			
1–2 p.m.			
2–3 p.m.			
3–4 p.m.			

4–5 p.m.			
5–6 p.m.			
6–7 p.m.			
7–8 p.m.			
8–9 p.m.			
9 p.m.–midnight			

COGNITION

In terms of cognition in depression, the client's thoughts can be negative and often self-blaming and self-critical. There can be a negative view of the world and the future.[11] Refer back to Chapters 3 and 4 for information about CBT. You will recall that the steps involved in CBT include:

- keeping a thought diary (to raise awareness)
- understanding unhelpful thinking patterns (such as 'catastrophizing')
- identifying unhelpful thinking
- challenging unhelpful thinking
- developing more helpful thoughts.

It is important to follow these five steps, one at a time, and it will take a number of sessions to work through them. To raise awareness of thinking (**step 1**), encourage the client to keep a thought diary, using the pro forma which follows on the next page. The client completes the date, and answers, 'What are you doing, how do you feel, and what are you thinking?'

Table 17: Thought diary

Date	What are you doing?	How do you feel? (name feeling and rate on a scale of 0–10)	What are you thinking?

For **step 2**, take the client through common unhelpful thinking patterns (see p. 51) so that they have a good understanding of them. **Step 3** involves asking the client to complete the next column relating to these in the pro forma below (Table 18), and **step 4** involves challenging the unhelpful thinking. Table 18 provides some examples of unhelpful thinking in depression, and also examples of more helpful ways of thinking.[12] This table can assist the counsellor in guiding the client to challenge their thinking, and to develop more helpful ways of thinking (**step 5**).

Table 18: Unhelpful thinking patterns and alternatives

Common unhelpful thinking patterns in depression	More helpful ways of thinking
All-or-nothing or black-and-white thinking: 'I'll never be able to manage', 'I have to get top marks'	Encourage the client to change their perspective by considering other possibilities, such as 'I might have some trouble managing, but I can cope', or 'I don't have to be perfect'.
Over-generalization: 'I always mess things up', 'I never get it right'	Help the client look for evidence to disprove their thinking — think about the times they did 'get it right', or ask other people what they think. What are the facts?
Labelling: 'I'm hopeless'	Encourage the client to avoid labels and to use different words such as, 'There are things I did well today, and I will work on the things that I want to do better'.
Catastrophizing: 'It's a disaster', 'What if I never meet anyone else?'	Work on a more balanced outlook — there is no reason to think the worst is likely to happen. The client can ask themselves what the most likely outcome is going to be. Questions like, 'Is it the end of the world?' or 'Am I exaggerating?' can be helpful. Avoid 'what ifs' — consider that something might be possible, but not actually probable.
Disqualifying the positives: 'They implied that I could have done better'	Check whether the client is discounting positive aspects of a situation. They can ask themselves, 'Am I only considering the negatives?'
Personalization: 'It must be my fault'	The client can ask, 'Am I blaming myself for things that are not my fault?' Avoid inflexible words such as 'must'.

The client can practise developing more helpful thinking patterns by completing the pro forma (see 'Managing negative thinking' pro forma, p. 297), which includes additional columns for 'unhelpful thinking patterns' and 'more helpful thoughts'. The client is also asked to reflect on how they feel following the more helpful thinking.

BELIEFS

In terms of CBT to manage depression, let's take the discussion to another level. Underlying beliefs that can influence our thinking were previously referred to. Beliefs or taken-for-granted ideas can operate at an unconscious level but come into play when we need to respond to situations. Just as you have helped the client learn to identify automatic thoughts, you can help them learn to identify underlying beliefs. In depression, they tend to be negative. They can relate to needing to be loved by everyone or needing to be 100 per cent successful or else be considered a failure. Just as the client learns to develop more helpful thinking patterns, the counsellor can guide them to become more aware of the beliefs influencing their thinking.

The table on p. 132 lists a number of unhelpful beliefs and gives alternative, more helpful views. Take the client through these and see if any of the beliefs resonate with them. Some may also be identified during therapeutic conversations, or through the thought diary.

Table 19: Unhelpful beliefs and alternatives[13]

Unhelpful beliefs	More helpful view
'All significant people in my life must love me and approve of me.'	'I would prefer to be liked by people but there is no way I can guarantee it.'
'I must always be competent, adequate and achieving in every area of my life.'	'No one can be like that all the time — I accept my strengths and weaknesses.'
'My life should progress easily and smoothly. Things should work out the way I want them to. It's awful when things go wrong.'	'Things are not necessarily going to go as I want. I will do my best to overcome obstacles, but if that isn't possible I will accept their existence.'
'My life experiences determine how I feel. How can I feel good when things don't go as they should?'	'Depending on how you view the world, individuals can be sad or disappointed.'
'It is better not to take risks, because when you stick your neck out, you can get easily hurt.'	'If you don't take sensible risks you will never know whether something is enjoyable or not. See uncertainty as a challenge.'
'I must always be in control of situations.'	'The world is full of chance, but life can be enjoyed despite this. Wanting perfect control leads to a sense of loss of control.'
'People should be sensitive to my needs and do what I believe is right.'	'People's sensitivity varies greatly, and they are generally looking after their own interests. I can be assertive about my needs.'
'The world should be a fair place. I must always be treated fairly.'	'I would prefer it were fair, but there is injustice in the world. I will do my best to encourage fairness but accept that it often won't be fair.'

The 'downward arrow' technique

The downward arrow technique can also assist the counsellor and client to take a thought and explore it for underlying beliefs. A thought is identified, and then the counsellor asks the client: 'What does this say or mean about you?' The counsellor repeats this question until the heart of the issue is identified. An example is provided in Figure 9.

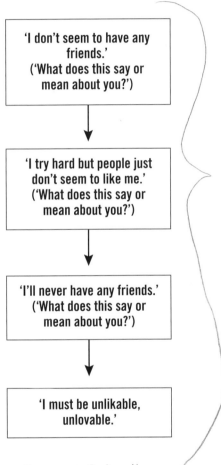

Figure 9: The downward arrow technique[14]

Once aware of unhelpful beliefs, the process of challenging and developing more helpful views can occur. The client might make a list of its **advantages and disadvantages** of the belief, to find the disadvantages outweigh the advantages. Another way of thinking about this is to weigh up how the belief works for them and how it works against them. The counsellor can then guide the client to challenge the unhelpful thinking relating to these beliefs. For example, with procrastination, the counsellor might ask the client: 'How does procrastinating, caused by believing that you must always do a fantastic job, work for you? How does it work against you?' No doubt it has advantages, but the stress caused and resultant, self-punishing self-talk and low mood may outweigh any of these.

Counsellors might be interested in further training in CBT, or in **Schema Therapy**, which focuses on exploring and identifying the client's beliefs about themselves, their relationship with others and their relationship with the wider environment. What are termed 'maladaptive coping schemas' can affect the client's expectations of themselves and their self-confidence, how they relate to others, their sense of pleasure and relaxation. There are questionnaires, such as the Young Schema Questionnaire, that identifies the schemas, which can then be addressed (refer to www.schematherapy.org).

PERFECTIONISM

It is also worth talking about perfectionism in this section, as perfectionistic tendencies can be involved in disappointment and depression. Perfectionism refers to wanting to do things extremely well, and it can result in the person putting pressure on themselves to meet high standards. Perfectionism can be viewed as a 'friend' by the client, helping them do a good job and be productive, or it can be viewed as a 'foe', as it is really an illusion (perfection is not actually possible). The underlying beliefs that can be involved in perfectionism include needing approval from others and to be 100 per cent competent in life, and needing to feel in control. These beliefs lead to traps in our thinking, such as all-or-nothing thinking, for example: 'If I don't do really well with this task, then it is not worth doing' or 'I must do things perfectly and never fail!' These patterns also lead to self-critical thinking, and perfectionists can define their self-worth by how well they perform.

LLCC TIP

Perfectionism can be helpful in life, but can also be a trap, leading to disappointment and depression. Learn to identify it with your clients and guide them on some ways to manage it.

Striving for an unrealistic level of perfection can cause stress and disappointment. It can also mean not delegating tasks that should be delegated, not starting or finishing a task, or a client never being satisfied with their performance. It can lead to procrastination, hoarding, difficulties making decisions, reassurance seeking, checking and avoidance of activities. So the message is that there is a big difference between healthily striving to do a good job and the unhelpful striving for perfection.

To identify perfectionism, ask the client:

- 'Do you have a need to do things right the first time, or think that you must do everything well?'
- 'Do you think there is no point in trying if you can't do it perfectly, or rarely give yourself credit for what you do?'
- 'Does your perfectionism prevent you from completing your work or other duties?'

If the client responds 'yes' to some of these questions, then some work on reducing perfectionism may be helpful.[15]

It may be helpful to take the client through some tips on how to be less of a perfectionist.

LLCC TIPS: DEALING WITH PERFECTIONISM

Remind the client to be aware of the following points.

- Be aware of expectations — one's own and others. Question whether they are realistic.
- Doing things perfectly does not necessarily make others see a person as more valuable or worthy of approval. It can also be very tiring.
- Weigh up the advantages and disadvantages of being a perfectionist. The client may want to keep some of the advantages, but let go of some of the disadvantages.
- As an experiment, the counsellor might encourage the person to sometimes lower their standards, for example, aiming to do a good job instead of a perfect job. Frustration and procrastination are likely to decrease, and the client might find that satisfaction increases. There will be more time to relax, too.
- Sometimes the client needs to put some limits on what they do, in terms of time spent on a task, for example.
- Encourage the client to be aware of any fear that might hide behind perfectionism, such as fear of failure or

criticism. Fear can maintain behaviours, and the way to deal with it is to challenge it.

■ Encourage them to recognize that change is always possible, and to keep things in perspective.

■ Make use of some questions to challenge thinking around being perfect. Examples might be:
   — 'Who says that I must always be perfect?'
   — 'What would happen if I made a mistake occasionally?'
   — 'Would it be the end of the world?'
   — 'What is the worst that could happen?'
   — 'Would that be so terrible? Could I live with that?'
■ Remember, very few things are perfect. It is okay to be average.[16]

PROCRASTINATION

Tied in with perfectionism is procrastination, or putting things off, which is a form of avoidant behaviour. Procrastination might be used to avoid a stressful situation, such as a student procrastinating over their assignments and handing them in late as a result. Sometimes using distractions, such as going on the Internet, watching movies or smoking, is a form of procrastination and the distractions can help to avoid uncomfortable feelings. It is important to weigh up whether distraction comes at a cost. It is also important for the client to be honest with themself and ask whether or not the avoidance is necessary. Another example of procrastination is delaying working on goals, such as exercising. Adopting different behaviours can assist, including setting realistic goals and breaking them down into small steps, with realistic timeframes.

Procrastination can be related to having high expectations of oneself. For example, an individual may procrastinate and be late with a piece of work because they want it to be perfect. Procrastination may also stem from fear of failure or criticism, a fear of uncertainty, a desire to be approved of by important people in your life or a desire to be in control of things. Sometimes it is related to self-doubt. In the case of a client expecting a lot of themselves, they need to challenge their thoughts and beliefs in relation to these expectations, and develop new perspectives on themself. In terms of wanting to be in control or fear of uncertainty, the client needs to challenge some of ideas about control, as life does involve uncertainty.

Key in managing procrastination is learning to sit with uncomfortable feelings, and mindfulness and ACT strategies can assist with this.[17]

> ## LLCC TIP
> Procrastination can relate to avoidance of uncomfortable feelings or high expectations of oneself. Encourage the client to set realistic goals, and to learn to sit with discomfort — ACT strategies can assist.

Mindfulness-based Cognitive Therapy

Some of the main research in relation to MBCT and depression is related to an eight-week group therapy program originally developed by Segal et al.[18] Research has found that this program significantly reduces depression relapse rates.[19] Manicavasagar et al. also found increased levels of mindfulness and lower levels of rumination following MBCT.[20] The principles and content of this program can be applied when working with individuals or in groups.

The core aims of MBCT are to help clients:

■ who have experienced depression in the past to learn skills to help prevent depression returning

■ to become more aware of bodily sensations, feelings and thoughts from moment to moment

■ to develop a different way of relating to sensations, thoughts and feelings, that is, through mindful acceptance and acknowledgement of unwanted feelings and thoughts, rather than habitual, automatic responses.

Initially an assessment is carried out, to learn about the factors that have for the client been associated with the onset and maintenance of depression, and to explain the background of MBCT and ensure the client is not acutely unwell.[21] The content of the MBCT group program includes:

■ **mindfulness skills** — basic mindfulness practices are undertaken, such as mindfully eating a sultana (noticing its smell, taste, texture), therapist-led body scan, or breathing mindfully; the focus is on experiencing the moment without becoming attached, aversive or bored

■ skills to manage negative mood shifts, with the goal of cultivating sustained wellness and protection from relapse; awareness of negative thoughts and fostering self-compassion are seen as keys to the program.

■ homework tasks between classes.[22]

The full MBCT program aiming to prevent depression relapse can be found in Segal, 2002 (see 'Resources' p. 150). A workbook on the program is now available for the public.

Acceptance and Commitment Therapy

ACT can be applied in depression. It highlights that even the language the counsellor and client use is important; for example, saying 'I am depressed' results in the client having a new story about themselves, and a new sense of self as being depressed. This storytelling can get in the way of psychological flexibility. In depression, the person can also become fused with thoughts about the past. ACT suggests that a sense of dysphoria develops, and the depression is avoidance of dysphoria; and trying to avoid depressive thoughts often leads to more depressive thoughts, as we have a tendency to focus on negative thoughts as part of our survival mechanisms. Rumination occurs in an attempt to regain what has been lost, and can lead to rigidity in thinking. Sometimes the client manages these issues with self-medication or self-harm.

According to ACT, the pathological processes in depression include:
- fusion with thoughts and feelings — managed with **defusion**
- experiential avoidance — managed with **acceptance**
- rumination — managed with **mindfulness**
- attachment to a damaged self-concept — management involves **self-as-context**.[23]

In addition, commitment and behaviour change are necessary. Motivational Interviewing and values-based goal setting may be utilized, and strengths are highlighted and barriers to recovery explored.

LLCC TIP
The following story from Japan can be helpful to share with clients; it demonstrates that emotions come and go, and can lead into discussion about acceptance.

Two men who know each other run into one another. 'How are you today?' asks the first man. The second replies, 'I am feeling good, thank you.' 'That will pass,' replies the first man. The men run into each other on another day, and again the first man asks, 'How are you today?' The other man replies, 'I am feeling very tired and low today.' The first man again responds, 'That will pass.'

A number of ACT interventions were described in Chapter 5 in relation to managing anxiety, and they are also helpful in depression (in particular, defusion techniques for troublesome thoughts, and the 'Being with an emotion' exercise found on p. 106). Several examples of additional ACT interventions to consider in managing depression follow:

- The **compass metaphor** highlights values and goals. This is based on the idea that a compass gives a person direction and keeps them on track. Values do the same in life.[24]

- **Mindfulness** exercises (see p. 103).

- The **tug-of-war with a monster metaphor** illustrates that there is a sense of struggle with depression, and sometimes we need to reduce our sense of struggle. The client is asked to imagine they are in a tug-of-war with a depression monster. They have one end of the rope and the monster has the other, and there is a pit in the middle. The client is asked what they need to do to prevent falling into the pit. The answer is not to pull harder, but to drop the rope or the struggle.[25]

- The **chess metaphor** can be utilized to discuss the role of self-as-context, defusion and action:

A chess match is like a war fought out between different armies of coloured pieces. The goal is for the white pieces to get rid of the black pieces and vice versa. For a moment, imagine a chess board that is infinitely large, extending out in all directions. There are thousands of pieces, and they band together and fight. Think of your thoughts, feelings, memories and beliefs as the white pieces on the board. You might like some of these pleasant memories you have accumulated . . . but there are black pieces too; think of them as depressing thoughts or negative feelings.

Remember, the black and white pieces battle each other. Be honest with yourself: don't you want the white pieces to win? You therefore have a stake in it, and maybe you often were drawn to the board to organize the white pieces against the black. Do the black pieces seem intimidating? As much as you try, given the board goes on and on, will you ever kick the black pieces you don't like off the board? To what degree has your struggle with depression been like fighting a war you haven't been able to win? Consider, too, that you might choose to be the board, rather than a player. It holds the pieces, and there is less stake in it. And the board can move forward.[26]

More information about ACT and depression can be found in the books about ACT highlighted in 'Resources' at the end of this chapter.

Interpersonal Therapy

IPT was originally developed for use in depression, and it poses the following questions:

1. What has contributed to the client's depression right now?
2. What are the current stresses?
3. Who are the key people involved in the current stresses? What are the current disputes and disappointments?
4. Is the client learning how to cope with the problem?
5. What are the client's strengths?
6. How can the counsellor help the client ventilate painful emotions — talk about situations that evoke guilt or shame or resentment?
7. How can the counsellor help the client clarify their wishes and have more satisfying relationships with others?
8. How can the counsellor correct misinformation and suggest alternatives?[27]

Attachment theory as outlined on page 40 is viewed as important in depression. The concept of attachment provides a theoretical basis for understanding the interpersonal context of depression, and for developing strategies to correct problems produced by impaired attachments in childhood.[28] A number of links between depression and attachment have been identified. For example: a disrupted or unloving relationship with a caregiver in childhood can predispose the client to depression; children of parents with depression are also more likely to suffer from depression; and persistent marital discord results in increased depression in children.[29]

Dealing with relationship issues through IPT can be a vital part of managing depression. A relationship breakdown may have contributed to the development of depression, or relationship problems might be causing ongoing stress. Perhaps there are problems in communicating, or maybe there are issues around intimacy with a partner. Depression itself, as well as any associated stress and anxiety, can cause fatigue and lower libido, and medication can sometimes have a negative effect. Whatever the issues, relationships often need some help. Giving time to a partner, listening and making an effort are important in a relationship, as well as showing interest in the other person and not criticizing. These can be challenging when depression is present, but small steps can be made at the start, and built upon over time.

LLCC TIP

When depression is present, pay attention to the client's relationships. The IPT timeline and inventory provide valuable information and insight.

IPT in depression will involve: *Interpersonal therapy*

- thorough assessment and formulation, including review of the symptoms, naming the problem as depression, and considering whether medication may be indicated (if so, it might be necessary to refer the client)
- providing **psycho-education** regarding depression and IPT
- carrying out an **interpersonal inventory** detailing current and past relationships with significant others, and a **timeline** (see p. 178)
- exploring the quality and patterns of interactions with others
- exploring the cognitions the client has developed about themselves and their relationships, including **expectations and meaning**
- considering whether any **unhelpful thinking patterns** are contributing to the relationship issues e.g. mind-reading between partners, being 'black and white', or catastrophizing
- establishing the **satisfying and unsatisfying** aspects of the client's main relationship, and whether the client wants changes in their relationship
- exploring associated **emotions** including pleasure, sadness, disappointment, anger, trust, fear, guilt, jealousy or shame[30]
- identifying major 'problem areas' related to the depression and setting management goals.

The counsellor will then focus on any of the four **problem areas** identified, and in working with these areas, the IPT techniques such as clarification and communication analysis (outlined on p. 109) are utilized. The four areas are as follows:

1. **Loss and grief.** It is important to identify any loss and grief and potentially relate these instances to the depression symptoms. In terms of managing grief, psycho-education about loss and grief, facilitating the mourning process and exploring the client's feelings are key (see Chapter 10 for grief counselling). Remember that situations such as job loss, and separation and divorce, are associated with loss and grief, and there are often feelings of hurt and anger to be worked through.[31]

2. **Transition.** This involves change, and it is important to identify associated losses (such as a particular role, family support or friendships)

and related mourning, and to work on highlighting the positive aspects of the new situation (see Chapter 11).

3. **Interpersonal disputes.** Any conflict relating to the depression is identified and explored. Strategies on conflict management outlined later in this chapter can then be utilized.

4. **Interpersonal sensitivities.** Identify any that relate to the depression, such as social isolation or difficulties relating to others. The aim will then be to reduce social isolation, encourage new relationships, and to teach new social skills. In depression there is a tendency to withdraw from people, and feeling lonely can be an issue. It is generally agreed that social connections play an important role in maintaining a sense of wellbeing. Loneliness is a form of disconnectedness, and feeling connected contributes to a sense of belonging.[32] It can be useful to explore the client's thinking; for example, they might think that 'no one cares', but maybe people have actually been helpful in the past and are perhaps unaware of the current problems.[33] Doing some goal-setting can assist, with the aim of becoming more active and involved with others.

Social skills training can be helpful in terms of managing depression, and it is often included in CBT and IPT approaches. We all need to be able to express ourselves assertively or directly at times. Clients may have difficulty expressing their opinion, or feel that their needs are not being met.

The following information on **assertiveness training** can be helpful in your work with clients. First, remind the client that assertiveness means being able to express your needs and feelings more directly. It involves changing the ways in which you relate to people and the behaviours that you use. Assertive and non-assertive behaviours are learnt. As children we are taught how to behave. For example, how did your family handle conflict? Being more assertive can be helpful in starting conversations, confronting others, dealing with annoyance, responding to criticism, turning down requests or asking for favours. In the long run, being more assertive also helps develop a greater sense of self-belief.[34] Second, inform the client that assertiveness is based on a number of rules and rights, namely: 'I have the right to respect myself, recognize my own needs as an individual, make clear "I" statements, allow myself to make mistakes, change my mind, ask for "thinking-over time", allow myself to enjoy my successes, ask for what I want, recognize that I am not responsible for the behaviour of other adults, and respect other people'.[35]

Table 20 summarizes three different types of behaviour: passive, assertive and aggressive.[36]

Table 20: Types of behaviour

Passive	Aggressive	Assertive
The client might:	The client might:	The client might:
■ avoid saying what they think or feel	■ offend others when they stand up for themselves	■ clearly communicate their feelings, thoughts and needs to others
■ avoid telling people what they want or would like	■ struggle to communicate effectively	■ avoid saying it doesn't matter when it does, in a tactful way
■ put other people's needs before their own	■ wait until they are really frustrated about something and then 'explode'	■ respect their own rights, but also those of others.
■ feel as if they are weak, inferior or incompetent.	■ talk over others and not let them have their say.	

There can be obstacles to being assertive, such as fear of offending the other person or worry that they won't approve. It is important for the client to remember that it is good to be sensitive to others, but that their rights are important too and they are not responsible for how the other person reacts. Being more assertive can impact on relationships. Other people might be used to interacting with the client in certain ways and can feel challenged when they become more assertive. Shyness, perfectionism and a belief in needing approval from everyone can be a barrier to being assertive, as can feelings of guilt.[37]

It is helpful for the client to learn how to use 'I' statements. These can explain:

■ the client's feelings about the person's behaviour or the effect of the behaviour ('I feel . . .')

■ what the unacceptable behaviour is in a non-blameful way ('When you . . .')

■ the effects of the behaviour on the client ('Because . . .')

■ what the client would like to happen ('I'd prefer . . .').[38,39]

Note that it is important for the client to also acknowledge the other person at the start of what they say. This means saying something like, 'I appreciate . . .' or 'I can see that you feel . . .'. Here is an example: 'I can see that you are feeling annoyed. However, I feel upset when you say "You're hopeless" because it affects my confidence. I want you to stop saying that, and recognize that I do a lot of things well.' The client also needs to be aware that as they speak assertively their tone should remain calm and steady, and their non-verbal communication be congruent with an upright and open posture, avoiding fidgeting and making eye contact. The key is to practise and to prepare for situations in which assertiveness may be necessary. The client might like to write down what they want to say and practise in front of the mirror at home, or with the counsellor.

Narrative Therapy

The following Narrative Therapy strategies can assist with depression.

- Discuss with the client the influences of society on them, the temptation to measure up to unrealistic ideals, and the impact of these influences on the client's sense of self-worth.
- **Externalize** the depression. That is, place the depression (the problem) outside of the person, and speak of how 'the depression' is affecting the client. Refer to how the client and their team (family, friends, counsellor etc.) can assist with managing the depression.
- Search for alternative experiences, as even during very difficult times people use their strengths and get through. Gradually build an **alternative story**.
- Use **narrative questioning** to explore the impact of the depression on the client's life and to draw out their strengths and exceptions to the depression. Refer back to page 111 and substitute the word 'depression' for 'anxiety' in the questions. For example, 'What is the impact of the depression on your life?', 'How has the depression impacted on your view of yourself?', and 'Think of a time when you have been able to stand up to the depression and stopped it pushing you around.'

LLCC TIP
Externalize the depression, and use narrative questioning to explore the impact of the depression on the client's life. Gradually build an alternative story.

Positive Therapy

Positive Therapy relates to fostering positive emotions, relationships and engagement in life. Early philosophers said that very little is needed to make a happy life, and a favourite quote by writer and poet Joseph Addison is that the 'three grand essentials to happiness in this life are something to do, something to love, and something to hope for'.[40] This quote illustrates Positive Therapy's application in depression; the approach encourages clients in the following ways:

- It helps the client identify their **values** and live according to them (see p. 33).
- It encourages the client to identify their **strengths** and use them more, whatever they may be (see p. 112).
- The fostering of **positive emotions** is encouraged, including kindness. When humans are kind to each other, uplifting hormones are released in the body, so the person being kind benefits as well as the recipient.

> **LLCC TIP**
> A kindness exercise might involve asking the client to perform one act of kindness a day, whether it be saying thank you, giving a compliment or making someone a cup of coffee.

- Positive Therapy suggests the client practise **gratitude**, which has been shown to be associated with positive emotions. Various gratitude exercises can be used, such as suggesting the client reflect on being thankful for the food they are eating that day, or once a week writing down three things they are grateful for. It may be appropriate for the client to start a ritual with their family, involving everyone naming something they are grateful for at a meal once a week.
- It urges the client to engage in leisure **activities**, initially through scheduling such activities into their week, and later through more engagement with them in day-to-day life (see p. 127). These can include creative activities, such as cooking or gardening. Adult colouring-in books are a popular creative (and mindful) activity.
- Clients are encouraged to tap into laughter and **humour** more as the depression improves. In depression it can be difficult to smile, let alone laugh. However, as the depression improves it becomes easier. There are many reasons to develop the ability to smile and laugh again: it helps general health and wellbeing; and laughter not only feels good due to endorphin release in the body, it is also relaxing.[41] Watching a comedy, funny clips on YouTube or reading a funny story can all assist.
- Practising **mindfulness**, everyday activities or meditation, is fostered.
- Engaging in social or work activities is also encouraged, as is building **social connections**.
- The client is assisted in developing social skills (such as listening to others, sharing feelings, being assertive).

- **Self-care** and **positive coping skills** are practised (such as problem-solving or developing helpful thinking patterns).
- It points the client towards focusing on **meaning** in life, through values and purpose. Accomplishing even small goals can assist.
- Developing **resilience** skills, which assist in reducing further impacts of the depression, is part of the Positive Therapy approach. This involves developing more flexibility in thinking and behaviours, focusing on the present and adopting a 'wait and see' attitude to the future. It also involves developing helpful coping mechanisms, such as problem-solving and helpful thinking.
- The client is aided in fostering **hope**, as it 'can be what sustains life in the face of despair'.[42] Counsellors can plant the seed of hope early on with depression, and continue to encourage connection with hope throughout recovery. Being supportive, normalizing symptoms and psycho-education play a part. Reading inspirational books and quotes can encourage and inspire. Fostering value-based activities, acceptance and narrative conversations can also assist. In particular, look for elements of the alternative story and view hope as a resource the client can draw upon. New Zealand counsellor Victoria Marsden has explored creative ways to hold onto hope between counselling sessions, such as having conversations about this concept, contemplating hope between sessions and acknowledging small steps made by the client.[43]

LLCC TIP

Fostering hope is vital. Plant the seed of hope early on, and continue to encourage hope throughout recovery. Inspirational stories and quotes can help.

Hypnotherapy

Hypnotherapy can be very helpful for a client experiencing depression. Note, however, that when the depression is severe, and cognition is affected, hypnotherapy is not appropriate as a level of concentration is required. As the client's mood and functioning improves, then hypnotherapy offers a number of helpful tools.

- Relaxation and **self-hypnosis** are helpful, especially when there are sleep disturbances or anxiety.
- Aspects of **psycho-education** can be repeated in the hypnotic state.

- **Direct suggestions** about feeling more calm, confident and positive each day can be utilized. Additionally, direct suggestions can be made about applying the various strategies the client has learnt to their everyday lives, such as lifestyle (eating healthily, exercising, getting adequate rest) and practising mindfulness.
- **Ego-strengthening** suggestions build self-belief, including reinforcing the client's strengths and reinforcing progress made each session.

LLCC TIP

Depression impacts significantly on self-confidence, and ego-strengthening suggestions in hypnosis are very useful. Focusing on strengths and progress, in and out of hypnosis, is powerful.

- Direct suggestions are used to **reinforce CBT**, such as suggestions about behavioural changes (including regular pleasant activities and relaxation) or reinforcing helpful thinking patterns versus unhelpful patterns, such as black-and-white thinking or labelling. Underlying beliefs, such as needing to be 100 per cent competent or approved of by everyone, can be challenged.
- Indirect suggestion or **metaphor** can also be used to encourage helpful thinking. Some years ago, a student I was teaching in a course on hypnosis, wrote a black-and-white metaphor, which spoke of a person going for a walk. At the start of the walk, everything around them was black and white. As they began to change their view of themselves and the world, it came to life in colour.
- The essence of the **ACT** model can be explained in the hypnotic state to reinforce understanding. Living a life consistent with values can be encouraged by asking the person in hypnosis to reflect on what is most important to them in life in the different domains. Being mindful can again be reinforced, and the concept of acceptance can be explored, as well as 'self-as-context' or the observing self. The various techniques can be reinforced and practised in the hypnotic state, and you will note that many of the ACT tools are hypnotic in nature, such as 'leaves on a stream' or 'Being with an emotion' (for more on ACT see pp. 103–107).
- Elements of **Narrative Therapy** can also be reinforced, such as externalizing the depression and the alternative story.
- **Self-compassion** (see Chapter 13) is encouraged through suggestions, either direct or indirect.

Bibliotherapy and e-mental health

Self-help Bibliotherapy is widely used in managing depression. There have been several meta-analyses (high-quality studies combining the results of other studies) suggesting that Bibliotherapy based on CBT is an effective treatment for depression.[44,45,46,47] There is also some evidence that creative Bibliotherapy (utilizing fiction) is helpful in reducing depression symptoms.[48] Books that describe other people's experiences of depression can be powerful in illustrating that the person is not alone in their experience of depression. Note that Bibliotherapy can only be utilized when the client is able to concentrate and has literacy skills.

I often utilize the following books in relation to depression:

- Howell, C. 2009, *Keeping the Blues Away: The ten-step guide to reducing the relapse of depression*, Radcliffe, London.
- Edelman, S. 2013, *Change Your Thinking: Positive and practical ways to overcome stress, negative emotions and self-defeating behaviour using CBT*, HarperCollins Publishers, Sydney.
- Harris, R. and Aisbett, B. 2013, *The Happiness Trap Pocketbook*, Exisle Publishing, New South Wales.

In terms of **e-mental health**, search 'depression' on the Beacon website (www.beacon.anu.edu.au), which reviews websites and online programs from around the world. Websites with useful materials for psycho-education include the websites for Australian organizations Beyondblue (www.beyondblue.org.au) and the Black Dog Institute (www.blackdoginstitute.org.au). For an online CBT-based program, the Australian National University has developed MoodGym, which can be found at http://moodgym.anu.edu.au.

In summary

Much of my working life has been involved in researching depression and relapse prevention, and assisting clients struggling with feelings of sadness or depression. My hope is that this section has provided useful information and inspiration to the reader. The essence of caring for a client experiencing sadness or depression is travelling with them, and so the therapeutic relationship is key. Guide the client, provide information, let them know that support is available and that there is hope. Encourage clients to care for themselves, to gradually re-engage with activity, and to be compassionate in their thinking about themselves. Much can be gained from the range of therapies outlined in this chapter.

Reflection on Taylor's story

Taylor was also assessed by her GP. Medication was thought to be necessary and Taylor agreed that to manage the demands of her course, it would be helpful. She was also found to be low in iron and was given iron supplements. Taylor's mother visited for a few weeks, and Taylor appreciated this support.

Taylor continued to see the counsellor regularly. She found the support and reassurance helpful. Working with the counsellor, Taylor decided to reduce her training for a couple of months to reduce the level of stress, and also worked on regulating her sleep.

Being more rested helped her cope with day-to-day activities. However, it became apparent over time that Taylor had not felt happy with the health course. She was worried about upsetting her parents, but with the counsellor's help she decided to defer her course and transfer into a related course the following semester. Her parents were supportive, and Taylor continued to improve.

LLCC TIPS: IMPROVING MOOD

- Get in touch with values and live them.
- Use inner strengths and resources.
- Connect with people.
- Be in the moment.
- Practise self-care, such as getting regular sleep and exercise, and healthy eating.
- Challenge unhelpful thinking and develop more optimistic thinking.
- Foster hope and acceptance.
- Remember the value of activity and humour — have a smile when able to.
- Appreciate others and the world.
- Practise kindness to others and oneself.

Resources

Books

Edelman, S. 2013, *Change Your Thinking: Positive and practical ways to overcome stress, negative emotions and self-defeating behaviour using CBT*, HarperCollins Publishers, Sydney.

Greenberger, D. and Padesky, C. 2016, *Mind Over Mood: Change how you feel by changing the way you think* (2nd ed.), Guilford Press, New York.

Harris, R. 2007, *The Happiness Trap: Stop struggling, start living*, Exisle Publishing, New South Wales.

Harris, R. 2009, *ACT Made Simple: An easy-to-read primer on Acceptance and Commitment Therapy*, New Harbinger Publications, California.

Harris, R. and Aisbett, B. 2013, *The Happiness Trap Pocketbook*, Exisle Publishing, New South Wales.

Howell, C. 2009, *Keeping the Blues Away: The ten-step guide to reducing the relapse of depression*, Radcliffe, London.

Howell, C. 2014, *Meditation and Mindfulness: What's all the fuss about?* e-book available at www.drcatehowell.com.au

McKenzie, S. and Hassed, C. 2012, *Mindfulness for Life*, Exisle Publishing, New South Wales.

Strohsahl, K. and Robenson, P. 2008, *The Mindfulness and Acceptance Workbook for Depression*, New Harbinger Publications, California.

Tanner, S. and Ball, J. 2012, *Beating the Blues: A self-help approach to overcoming depression*, Doubleday, Sydney.

Teasdale, J. Williams, M. and Segal, Z. 2014, *The Mindful Way Workbook: An 8-week program to free yourself from depression and emotional distress*, The Guilford Press, New York.

Young, J. and Klosko, J. 1993, *Reinventing Your Life: The breakthrough program to end negative behaviour . . . and feel great again*, Plume, New York.

Zettle, R. 2007, *ACT for Depression: A clinician's guide to using ACT in treating depression*, New Harbinger Publications, California.

Websites

ACT and mindfulness: www.actmindfully.com.au

Beyondblue: www.beyondblue.org.au

Black Dog Institute: www.blackdoginstitute.org.au/public/research/ehealth.cfm

Blue Pages depression information: www.bluepages.anu.edu.au

Centre for Clinical Interventions: www.cci.health.wa.gov.au

MoodGym Online treatment program for depression (CBT): https://moodgym.anu.edu.au

New Zealand mental health resources: www.mentalhealth.org.nz/get-help/a-z

Royal Australian and New Zealand College of Psychiatrists: www.ranzcp.org

South African Depression and Anxiety group: http://www.sadag.org/

Youth Beyondblue: www.youthbeyondblue.com

Phone apps

Smiling Mind: www.smilingmind.com.au

Optimism apps: www.findingoptimism.com

Chapter 7
Taming anger

Raise your words, not voice. It is rain that grows flowers, not thunder.

—RUMI

The emotion of anger is a strong and often uncomfortable emotional reaction to another person or event. It occurs when our beliefs about the way things should be in a particular situation are contradicted.[1] Anger ranges from irritation to rage. When we think of anger, we often think of it in a negative light. Certainly, anger can lead to many destructive behaviours, such as aggression or substance use, but it is important to remember that it is a normal response to many situations. Anger can let us know when something is wrong. In fact, our survival at times may rely on us going into 'fight' mode. Anger can energize us, or motivate us to communicate more or to make positive changes in life.

Clients may present with issues related to anger, or anger might become an apparent issue as the counsellor hears the story. This section will focus on strategies for understanding and managing destructive anger. Consider Robert's and Samantha's stories, and as you read about anger reflect on the approaches which might assist them.

Robert's story

Robert, 35 years old, lives alone. He has had some health issues and has struggled with depression and anxiety for several years. He has used substances in the past, but now is on medication for the depression and is not using any recreational drugs. He is not able to work at present, and struggles intermittently with feelings of anger. The feelings of depression and anger can be overwhelming and have resulted in Robert withdrawing from people, in part due to fears that he will get into physical confrontations with others.

Samantha's story

Samantha, who is 29 years old, works in recruitment and lives with her partner Rob. She presents for help with stress management, and tells the counsellor that her job is stressful, that she and Rob are having some difficulties, and that she is perceiving her parents want her to settle down and have children. She is irritable with people and starting to lose her temper at home and at work. Anger was rarely expressed in her family growing up, and Samantha thinks that she should be able to control her angry feelings. She struggles to be assertive and express to others what she thinks.

Background

Consider how the 'umbrella of life' influences men's and women's views on and expression of anger. Robert and Samantha, for example, might have had quite different influences in relation to anger growing up, causing them to think about and express their anger differently. Samantha, for example, might have grown up with anger being viewed as 'bad', and something not to be expressed. Robert might have learnt that expressing anger physically was acceptable or a way to survive bullying.

A few points to remember:

- Anger is neither good nor bad; it is a normal emotion and can be a healthy **motivator**.
- Anger issues can be explored with clients in individual counselling or in group settings.
- Everyone feels and expresses anger differently — some clients will internalize anger and others will deal with it at the time.

- There are several ways clients can experience anger, namely:
  - **behavioural** anger, such as crying, shouting, shoving and hitting
  - **cognitive** anger, that is, thoughts or images, often exaggerated
  - **physiological** anger, including breathing, heart rate, flushed face or sweating.[2]

LLCC TIP

Help the client identify how they experience anger (with behaviours, thoughts, physical sensations). Explain that the physical symptoms are much like the fight or flight response.

Sometimes myths that a client develops need to be dispelled, such as 'I cannot control my anger' or 'I will explode unless I let it out'.

Cognitive Behaviour Therapy

CBT is very helpful for clients in learning to understand and modify angry reactions. Explain to the client the CBT cycle (see p. 50), and that the angry feelings are associated with thoughts and behaviours. Explore a range of questions with them to aid understanding. Such questions could include the following:

- 'Are there any particular events or situations that trigger feelings of anger?'
- 'What are the signs in your body that let you know you are becoming angry (such as feeling hot, muscle tension, palpitations or sweating)?'
- 'Is the anger related to something you expected to happen, or you expected from another person?'
- 'Are the feelings of anger associated with other feelings such as shame, hurt, guilt or fear?'
- 'Do you express your anger/how do you generally express your anger?'

LLCC TIP

It can be helpful to take a recent incident in relation to anger and explore these questions in relation to that incident.

Spend time on the **cognitive** aspect of CBT, as there might be unhelpful thinking patterns associated with the anger, examples being black-and-white thinking and catastrophizing. The steps outlined on page 128 can be helpful in raising awareness of thinking, and to identify unhelpful thinking patterns and challenge and reframe these. Some of the underlying beliefs the client holds, such as 'The world should be fair' or 'Bad things shouldn't happen', may influence the emotion of anger. Again, awareness of and challenging these beliefs can assist. The counsellor needs to listen for the client consistently placing blame outside of themselves; sometimes this might be justified and at other times not.

LLCC TIP

Keeping an anger journal can be helpful in raising awareness. The journal·can include

- events and triggers
- feelings rated from 0 to 10 in intensity
- thoughts when feeling angry
- physical feelings
- any behaviours, such as throwing something or eating
- how long the anger lasted.

Problem-solving

Problem-solving can assist once the triggers for anger are understood. If the trigger is a repeating interaction in a relationship, explore with the client other ways to approach it, such as the client preparing what they want to say, and talking with the person when calm. If stress is contributing to the anger, then stress management may be important, or if the client is struggling with self-belief and security in a relationship, for example, then working on this may assist (see Chapter 13).

A useful tool in managing angry feelings comes from Chapter 2 of Petracek's *The Anger Workbook for Women*. Dealing with angry feelings is said to involve a three-part process: recognising the feelings; owning the feelings; responding to the feelings. This process acknowledges that anger warrants expression, but the client has the choice of how, when and where to express it. Delaying (by counting one to ten and walking away) and expressing it when calm can be a useful choice. Distraction can assist at times. This model also acknowledges that individuals need to own their own feelings in order to prevent blaming others or building up resentment over time.[3]

LLCC TIP

The metaphor of a set of traffic lights is helpful in anger and reflects Petracek's three-step process. Red represents recognizing triggers and the angry feelings (including the physical sensations); orange involves owning the feelings and taking some time (maybe taking a few breaths); green represents responding in helpful ways.

Acceptance and Commitment Therapy

The ACT model is applicable when the client is experiencing difficulties with anger. Assisting the client to be aware of their values, and how anger fits (or not) with these values is a helpful starting point. Useful skills in managing anger stem from:

- **mindfulness**, or contact with the present moment — to raise awareness of the anger and associated physical sensations and thoughts; being mindful of the breath is a helpful way to sit with the feelings and take some time before responding
- **defusion** of feelings and thoughts, to deal with the discomfort of the emotion and to defuse potentially unhelpful thoughts
- **acceptance** of uncomfortable feelings and thoughts and the difficult things in life, to assist with the sense that 'It is not fair and shouldn't happen'.
- **self-as-context** (the part of the mind that notices thoughts and feelings, that is calm and non-judgmental) – to assist with making a helpful choice about how to respond to the angry feelings or thoughts
- committed **action**, to encourage taking action such as taking time out and calming down, or expressing the anger constructively.

NAME YOUR FEELINGS

A useful ACT exercise for managing anger is **NAME your feelings** — **n**otice, **a**cknowledge, **m**ake space, **e**xpand awareness. Encourage the client to find a comfortable place to sit down and practise the following steps in order:

- **Notice**. 'Take several breaths in and out and notice the feel of the air as it flows through the nostrils and down into the lungs, and out again. You can add words such as, 'letting go' as you breathe out. Now move your awareness to your body: where is the feeling of anger strongest? Scan from head to toe. Notice as much as you can — how warm or heavy is the feeling? Is it prickly or hard? What colour is it?'

■ **Acknowledge**. 'Say to yourself "Here's a feeling of anger" rather than "I'm angry" because you are *not* your emotions. Or use just one word, such as "anger".'

■ **Make space**. 'Now breathe in deeply, and imagine your breath flows into and around that feeling in your body. As it does, notice that a space opens up inside you. Give the feeling permission to be there, maybe saying "opening up" and make peace with the feeling. Keep breathing like this, opening up gradually.'

■ **Expand awareness**. 'Now it's time to connect with the world around you. Where are you, what are you doing, who are you with? What can you see, hear and touch? Ask yourself, "What would I like to do now that's consistent with my values?"'

Initially the client will need to practise this set of steps every day, doing a brief version (30 seconds to 1 minute) five to ten times a day to start with when feeling stressed or irritated. They will gradually practise for longer periods, and with practice they will be able to do the NAME exercise when anger is present, such as during an argument.

ACCEPTANCE TOOL KIT

The **acceptance tool kit** described in Harris involves a script for various techniques to assist the process of acceptance, including observing the body and noticing where the feeling (such as anger) is located, observing the feeling, breathing into it, allowing it to be there, objectifying it (shape, size, colour), normalizing the feeling (i.e. recognizing it is giving the client information) and expanding awareness. The full script is available in *ACT Made Simple: An easy-to-read primer on Acceptance and Commitment Therapy* by Dr Russ Harris.

LLCC TIP

Discuss with the client the *Serenity prayer* by Reinhold Niebuhr, which focuses on acceptance. The counsellor should be aware of the client's beliefs, and can adapt the prayer as appropriate, such as leaving in or removing the word God or referring to it as a verse. The prayer has such an inherently powerful message, it can be very helpful in the counselling setting.

> *God, grant me the serenity to accept the things I cannot change;*
> *The courage to change the things I can;*
> *And the wisdom to know the difference.*

Narrative Therapy

The influence of socialization on the ways men and women experience anger has already been touched upon. This can be explored in relation to the client, and the messages they have taken on board from their family, school, media and culture, for example. Women, for example, might have learnt that anger is unacceptable and to internalize any angry feelings. The client might not have awareness of their emotions, might have learnt to put others' feelings before their own or actually deny feeling angry. As a result they may hold onto resentment, stay angry for longer, or direct it at themselves through overeating or self-harming behaviours, for example. Men might be more comfortable with constructively expressing feelings of anger, such as through sporting activities, or they might have learnt to express it destructively through their physicality, or by blaming or sulking when angry. Both men and women may fear their own anger.[4]

Narrative Therapy encourages conversations about anger. Applying narrative questioning to anger can assist in raising awareness (see pp. 111–112), for example, 'What is the impact of anger on your life? or 'How has anger impacted on your view of yourself?'. Look for exceptions to destructive anger, exploring whether there have been times when the client has constructively expressed their anger. In this way an alternative story can gradually be built. A narrative approach also enables discussion about responsibility for the anger and how it is responded to. An event or the actions of a person might have triggered feelings in the individual, but blaming is not always appropriate. Taking responsibility is particularly relevant when there is **domestic violence**. The counsellor needs to be clear with the client about what is acceptable and unacceptable in terms of behaviour. Using conversation to encourage awareness, particularly of the impact of destructive behaviours on others, is vital.

Interpersonal Therapy

In relationships, anger is often related to expectations not being met. IPT encourages the client to:

- consider how realistic their expectations are and whether they have been clearly communicated to the other person
- practise **communication and assertiveness** skills
- learn **conflict management** skills
- learn how to set **boundaries** with others where appropriate, for example, when the client is not being treated with respect by someone in their family or at work.

The following points can aid conflict management. Many arguments stem from differences in values or personality. Identifying the cause of the conflict, learning to compromise, accept and respect differences is central. Naming the conflict story can be also helpful when there is recurrent conflict over the same theme, such as the 'housework story' or the 'money story'. Use humour, avoid the 'I'm totally right and you're totally wrong story', and let go of the need to have the last word![5] Anger is a fact of life. Problems arise when there is escalation of anger through criticism, defensiveness, contempt or shutting down.[6]

LLCC TIP
Ask the client to spend time working through the conflict with the other person, by listening. The issue is highlighted, and then each person involved in the conflict talks about it, uninterrupted for 10 to 15 minutes. There is no attempt to solve the issue — the aim is understanding the other's perspective.[7]

Talk with clients about the tactics they use in arguments, such as springing conflict on the other person, or generalizing the discussion to things in the past. There are various ground rules for **fair fighting** which can be used.

- Beforehand, ask yourself why you feel upset.
- Discuss one issue at a time, and stay with the topic.
- Do not use degrading language.
- Express feelings in words and take responsibility for them, for example, 'I feel angry [or hurt etc.]'.
- Avoid stonewalling.
- Avoid yelling.

- Take time out if need be.
- Attempt to come to a compromise.[8]

Problem-solving can assist with some conflicts. Others are more perpetual, and acceptance of differences is required. Even when the problem cannot be solved, each person can learn to soothe the other person.

Hypnotherapy

Hypnotherapy can be helpful when there are issues with anger, through relaxation and **self-hypnosis** skills, reinforcing **mindfulness** skills, and the use of **ego-strengthening** suggestions to build self-belief.

Direct suggestions can be made about handling those situations that previously led to destructive anger, in more helpful ways. Direct suggestions can also be utilized regarding the specific techniques the client will use, for example, employing the traffic light metaphor to recognize and own their anger and respond constructively (see p. 156). Suggestions reinforcing the principles and strategies of **CBT** and client success can also be made in Hypnotherapy.

Situations that might trigger anger, such as particular interactions, can be **mentally rehearsed** as can various techniques to manage these situations.

Indirect suggestions such as metaphors can be used. Examples include the following two stories:

- There is a young boxer who not only gets into fights in the ring, but also outside the ring. As a result, his boxing career is in jeopardy, so his trainer teaches him to manage his fighting instinct in three different ways [insert the three most appropriate strategies for the client] in order to contain the fighting instinct when required.
- A 'storm watcher' follows storms around the country, observing storms brewing, building, coming to a crescendo with lightning and thunder, followed by calm. Some storms are major storms and others smaller and very brief. The storm watcher always watches the storms from a place of safety and does not get caught up in them. They accept that the storms will come, and they will go. Each is just a storm that will pass in time.

THE ANGER ROCK

Helen Watkins developed a hypnotic technique called the **anger rock**. This is a psychodynamic technique for those skilled in hypnotherapy, and it can be a valuable tool for clients to safely release anger while in the relaxed state.

When doing this sort of work, a safe place in the imagination is always set up. The nature of this will vary between clients, but can be a house or a place in the countryside, for example. Once the client has chosen a suitable safe place, begin the exercise, as in the script below.

> *Now you're going to walk from your safe place to a clearing, in the middle of which is a boulder. This boulder represents what it is you feel angry about right now. Next to the boulder is a mallet. Pick up the mallet and hit the boulder with it, as much or as little as you need to, to express your anger. Keep hitting the anger rock until you feel you are rid of the anger, then finish when you are ready.*

It is important to then focus the client on a positive experience, perhaps imagining relaxing in their safe place, and providing some positive suggestions about feeling calm and at peace.

Positive Therapy

Ideas from Positive Therapy can also assist with managing anger.

- The therapy utilizes the client's **values** and focuses on their **strengths**, which help them manage or constructively express angry feelings. Examples are being a good communicator or being able to creatively solve problems. With the client, look at how these strengths can assist in managing anger and encourage greater use of them.
- **Positive emotions** are fostered, including gratitude and kindness. Engagement in life also fosters positive emotions.
- **Leisure and creativity** (e.g. sport, music and art) can provide opportunities to express a range of emotions, including anger. Note that this also fits with expressive therapies (see p. 63).
- Positive Therapy helps build social and emotional skills for positive relationships, such as **communication and assertiveness skills**.
- Mindfulness, **self-care and positive coping skills**, such as problem-solving are encouraged (see p. 94)
- There is a focus on a sense of purpose and **meaning**, as well as building **resilience** skills (see p. 114).

Bibliotherapy and e-mental health

Some clients will engage well with **Bibliotherapy** in relation to anger. There are a number of good books about managing conflict or anger.

- Edelman, S. 2013, *Change Your Thinking: Positive and practical ways to overcome stress, negative emotions and self-defeating behaviour using CBT*, HarperCollins Publishers, Sydney.
- Eifert, G. and McKay, M. 2006, *ACT on Life Not on Anger: The new Acceptance*

and Commitment Therapy guide to problem anger, New Harbinger Publications, California.

- Lerner, H. (2014), *The Dance of Anger: A woman's guide to changing the patterns of intimate relationships*, HarperCollins Publishers, New York.
- Petracek, L. J. (2004), *The Anger Workbook for Women*, New Harbinger, California.

The modules on assertiveness written by the Centre for Clinical Interventions in Western Australia are excellent for **e-mental health**, and there is helpful information on both the British National Health Service and the American Psychological Association websites.

In summary

The emotion of anger will often arise in the counselling setting. It can be a strong and uncomfortable emotion for clients and counsellors. Anger is a normal response to many situations and can be very helpful, but it can also lead to destructive behaviours such as aggression or substance use. It is important to be aware that it can be part of depression or PTSD.

Many therapies and techniques can assist clients in managing anger. Reflect on Robert's and Samantha's stories and the range of strategies used.

Reflection on Robert's story

The counsellor undertook a thorough assessment with Robert. His mood had improved with medication, but he was still struggling with anxiety symptoms and anger. These emotions were explored, as were the situations in which they occurred and various triggers. It was found that Robert struggled with social anxiety, and his worst fear was becoming angry with others and embarrassing himself, or escalating the anger and potentially hurting someone. As a child he had seen his father get involved in physical altercations, and the link between this and his own fears was made.

The counsellor took Robert through CBT and ACT and the various strategies, in particular helping him recognize triggers to anxiety and anger, and learn to challenge unhelpful thinking. Robert found mindfulness meditation helpful and learnt to sit with discomfort and soothe himself. Assertiveness skills gave him more confidence in relating to others, and he was encouraged to gradually reengage with others. These skills were reinforced in hypnosis, and an anchor provided, as well as ego-strengthening.

Reflection on Samantha's story

Samantha and the counsellor explored some of the relationship issues via an interpersonal inventory. This created more insight into aspects of significant relationships which were generating stress, and which needed to be worked through.

Triggers to the anger were explored, along with ways to manage these triggers and the angry feelings. Samantha decided to go back to running regularly as a way of coping with stress. She found the traffic light metaphor particularly helpful, as well as taking some time out and the script for expressing herself more assertively.

Samantha was seen with her husband for a session to explore some of their issues in resolving conflict, and they were keen to try some of the strategies suggested.

LLCC TIPS: MANAGING ANGER

- Recognize triggers to anger.
- Don't bottle up frustrations; work out the cause of the anger, and communicate effectively about it.
- Let off steam through talking, exercise or creative expression such as music or art.
- Practise stress management techniques regularly.
- Don't sweat the small stuff. Pick life's battles, and remember there are some things that cannot be changed!
- Put the anger aside and deal with the problem instead.
- Be mindful of thinking patterns such black-and-white thinking or catastrophizing. Ask the question, 'Is it worth getting angry about?' and use calming thoughts, such as, 'Calm down, breathe and relax'.
- Recognize the warning signs of anger in the body, for example, muscle tension or teeth grinding.
- Take time out if feeling angry, and breathe, count to ten, tune into the senses or go for a quick walk.
- Remember your rights and the rights of others — to have an opinion, to be treated respectfully.
- Know personal troublesome angry behaviours, accept responsibility and work on them.
- Look for the positives in situations.

Resources

Books

Edelman, S. 2013, *Change Your Thinking: Positive and practical ways to overcome stress, negative emotions and self-defeating behaviour using CBT*, HarperCollins Publishers, Sydney.

Eifert, G. and McKay, M. 2006, *ACT on Life Not on Anger: The new Acceptance*

& Commitment therapy guide to problem anger, New Harbinger Publications, California.

Harris, R. 2007, *The Happiness Trap: Stop struggling, start living*, Exisle Publishing, New South Wales.

Harris, R. 2009, *ACT Made Simple: An easy-to-read primer on Acceptance and Commitment Therapy*, New Harbinger Publications, California.

Howell, C. 2009, *Keeping the Blues Away: The ten-step guide to reducing the relapse of depression*. Radcliffe, London.

Lerner, H. 2014, *The Dance of Anger: A woman's guide to changing the patterns of intimate relationships*. HarperCollins, New York.

Petracek, L.J. 2004, *The Anger Workbook for Women*, New Harbinger, California.

Websites

ACT Mindfully: www.actmindfully.com.au

Assertiveness: www.cci.health.wa.gov.au/

Beyondblue: www.beyondblue.org.au

Black Dog Institute: www.blackdoginstitute.org.au/public/research/ehealth. cfm

Phone apps

Breathe2Relax: t2health.dcoe.mil/apps/breathe2relax

Breathing Zone: www.breathing-zone.com

Meditation Oasis: www.meditationoasis.com

Smiling Mind: www.smilingmind.com.au

Chapter 8
Guilt and shame

Guilt and shame are normal emotions, which can surface in the counselling setting and potentially stem from a range of causes, such as past abuse or past behaviours, or in relation to body image, finances, parenting or relationships. Be aware that clients might be reluctant to raise or talk about guilt and shame, especially if there is perfectionism, because of the discomfort and vulnerability they cause.

Helen's story

Helen has been dealing with depressed feelings since the death of her husband, Rob, two years ago. He had cancer and she nursed him at home in the months before he died.

Helen has many friends and interests, but is struggling to engage with them. The counsellor notices that she often speaks critically about herself, and when the counsellor explores Helen's feelings it becomes apparent that the most troublesome ones are guilt and shame. Helen is holding on to a sense of guilt that she could have done more for Rob, and that sometimes she was grumpy with him in his final days, and she 'should not have been'.

Background

There has been more awareness of the place of shame and guilt in our lives following the publication of the work of renowned US researcher, Brené Brown. Brown defines shame as 'the intensely painful feeling or experience of believing that we are flawed and therefore unworthy of love and belonging'.[1] This results in fear of disconnection from others.[2] Brown says that guilt relates to the thought 'I did something bad', whereas shame relates to 'I am bad'. Brown also notes that shame triggers a fear of being unlovable. Shame and guilt might keep our behaviours in line, but shame is more likely to lead to self-destructive behaviours.[3] Based on the work of Hartling, Brown writes that in response to shame some people move away from it through silence or withdrawal; others move towards it by seeking to appease others; and still others try to move against it by gaining power over others. She says that all these 'move us away from our story' or sense of worthiness and embracing imperfections.[4] Rather, we need to recognize when we are experiencing shame so that we can act with intention.

Brown explores ways in which we can develop shame resilience, namely by:

- recognising shame and understanding its triggers
- reality-checking the messages and expectations that tell us that being imperfect means being inadequate
- reaching out and sharing our stories with people we trust
- talking about how you feel and asking for what you need.[5]

Brown writes about **vulnerability** — or showing our uncertainty, feelings or needs — as being at the core of a meaningful life. She says that being willing to engage with vulnerability involves risk and courage. The result, however, is that accessing vulnerability leads to trust and connection with self and others.[6] It can lead to a greater sense of safety and happiness.

LLCC TIP

Reflect on how the client can utilize Brown's 'enough' mandate:

- I am enough (that is, worthy).
- I've had enough (say no to one-upping and comparisons).
- I will show up, take risks, and let myself be seen.[7]

Cognitive Behaviour Therapy

CBT is very helpful for clients in learning to understand and manage feelings of guilt and shame. It is important that clients understand the CBT cycle, and how thoughts and underlying beliefs can influence the feelings of guilt and shame. There might be unhelpful thinking patterns associated with these feelings, such as mind-reading or labelling ('They think I am a bad person'). The steps outlined on page 98 can be helpful to raise awareness of thinking, to identify unhelpful thinking patterns and to challenge and reframe these. Some of the underlying beliefs the client holds, such as 'I should be 100 per cent competent' and 'approved of by everyone' can influence guilt and shame. Awareness and challenging these beliefs can assist.

Acceptance and Commitment Therapy

The ACT model is very applicable with guilt and shame. Assisting the client to become aware of their values, and if guilt and shame fit with these values or not, is a helpful starting point. Again, helpful skills in managing guilt and shame include:

- **mindfulness** or contact with the present moment — to raise awareness of the feelings and associated physical sensations and thoughts. Mindfulness of the breath is a helpful way to sit with the feelings and take some time before responding
- **defusion** of feelings and thoughts — to deal with the discomfort of the emotion and to defuse thoughts that may not be helping; the 'Being with an emotion' exercise as described on page 106 can be helpful
- **acceptance** of uncomfortable feelings and thoughts and the difficult things in life
- **self-as-context** or the observing mind to assist with making a helpful choice in how to respond to the feelings or thoughts
- committed **action** — to encourage taking action, such as expressing the feelings or practising thought defusion techniques.

The 'NAME your feelings' exercise utilizes the ACT processes and can assist with managing guilt and shame. It is important that the client practise the steps regularly, as below.

- **Notice**. 'Take several breaths in and out and notice the feel of the air as it flows in through your nostrils, and down into the lungs. You can add words such as, 'letting go' as you breathe out if you like. Now move your awareness to your body: where is the feeling (of guilt or shame) strongest? Scan from head to toe. Notice as much as you can — how warm or heavy is the feeling? Is it prickly or hard? What colour is it?'

- **Acknowledge**. 'Say to yourself "Here's a feeling of guilt (or shame)" rather than "I'm guilty (or ashamed)" because you are *not* your emotions. Or use just one word, such as "anger".'
- **Make space**. '**Now breathe in deeply, and imagine your breath flows into and around that feeling in your body. As it does, notice that a space opens up inside you. Give the feeling permission to be there, maybe saying "opening up" and make peace with the feeling.' Keep breathing like this, opening up gradually.'
- **Expand awareness**. 'Now it's time to connect with the world around you. Where are you, what are you doing, who are you with? What can you see, hear and touch? Ask yourself, "What would I like to do now that's consistent with my values?"'[8]

Interpersonal Therapy

IPT enables exploration of the client's story and relating emotions to life events. If relationships are part of the story of guilt and shame, then these can be explored. Problem areas such as associated loss and grief can be managed. Helen's story highlights the helpfulness of this approach (see the reflections on her story at the end of this chapter).

In relation to couples, infidelity may trigger guilt or shame (see Chapter 12). It is also important to be aware of the potential for childhood abuse or rape being part of the client's story (see Chapter 11).

Narrative Therapy

Revisiting the 'umbrella of society' with Narrative Therapy and how this might influence the client's beliefs or thoughts can be helpful. Have they developed unrealistic expectations about themselves? Discussing their 'humanness' is important. Being curious and having therapeutic conversations about guilt and shame can lead to more understanding and insight. Narrative questioning (see p. 111) can assist in raising the client's awareness about the impact of guilt and shame on their life. Highlighting the dominant story of guilt and shame and searching for the alternative story is part of this process. A narrative approach enables responsibility to be taken where needed, but also facilitates letting go of issues the client is not responsible for.

Expressive therapies

Expressive therapies can play a very useful role with guilt and shame. Practices such as art or drama can enable some clients to tap into those emotions and express them more readily than talking therapies. Examples are painting one's feelings, painting with music, or journalling about one's emotions.

Hypnotherapy

All of the previously discussed ideas and strategies can be reinforced through Hypnotherapy. There is also a useful hypnotic technique for releasing emotions. During hypnosis, a safe and peaceful place is established in the client's mind (for many this will be the beach, while for others it might be the countryside). If the client chooses a place near the water, establish an image of a boat; for the countryside, a hot air balloon. A script follows for the boat and balloon.

> *As you walk along the beach, notice there is a boat tethered to the shore. This is not a boat to go sailing in, but it is a special boat. On the sand nearby are some sponges, pieces of driftwood and cuttlefish. Gather a few of these up into your hands. Now each of these can represent something you would like to release, maybe an emotion or a troublesome thought.*
>
> *Take a few moments to reflect on what you wish to release, then attach each one to one of the items in your hands. One at a time, throw them into the boat. When all are in the boat, untie the rope and toss it into the boat as well. The boat will drift out over the waves, far away where what you have released will no longer be of any concern. You can always call your boat back to do more work if you wish to.*

If the client chooses the countryside, suggest that they come across a hot air balloon in a field, and that this is not a balloon to go flying in but a special balloon. Go on to say:

> *Notice any pattern on the balloon and the colours, and the basket suspended from the balloon. It is tethered to the ground by a rope. On the ground nearby there are some sticks, pine cones and stones. Gather a few up into your hands; each one represents something you would like to release. Attach meaning to each of the items in your hands and then, one at a time, throw them into the basket. Take your time, and when you have finished untie the balloon and it will float up, far far away where it need not be a concern. You can call the balloon back to do more work with it if you need to.*

At a workshop run by Helen Watkins many years ago, another technique was described for working with emotions. I have adapted it over the years, and it has proved very helpful for clients. It helps clarify which emotions are an issue for the client (often new insights develop) and it allows further processing of the emotions.

The counsellor explains to the client that they are going to take them through a technique to explore the current issues, and to see which emotions are most active. Ensure the client consents to this process. The counsellor then takes some pieces of paper and asks the client to tell them about the issue which is troubling them the most. They instruct the client that they will be writing down what the client says as they speak, and they will not interrupt them as they share the story. The client then tells the story of this issue uninterrupted, and the counsellor writes down all the words. If there seems to be a change in the topic or emotion described, the counsellor moves onto a new piece of paper.

Once the counsellor has checked that the client has finished sharing the story, the counsellor then reads back the story for the client. It usually becomes apparent that the story is broken into segments. These are then divided up — they may already be on different pieces of paper, but if on the same piece of paper they are cut apart. The segment or part of it is then read out loud by the counsellor and the client asked to give that segment a name, for example, 'mess' or 'despair' or 'anger'. Often the title is an emotion and if not, the client can also be asked if there are any emotions tied in with it.

The counsellor then lays each of the segments on the desk or table and asks the client to place them around the room, anywhere they like, and to go with their first response to this — they could be placed on or under furniture, for example. The client does this, and then the counsellor and client can discuss why they chose these spots. The place chosen often demonstrates how active the emotion is, and whether it has been dealt with. It might be kept close to the client or put in a rubbish bin, or filed away somewhere. Interesting insights are gained, and the client can often see that some segments are dealt with or need to be put away. The more active ones are to be worked on further in counselling.

In summary

Clients will at times struggle with these emotions of guilt and shame. They can be particularly distressing. It is important for the counsellor to listen carefully for any clues to guilt and shame, and have conversations with the client about them. Many of the strategies outlined can assist — as you read the reflection on Helen's story, identify which ones the counsellor utilized and consider which ones you might find helpful in your work. Also note that the therapeutic relationship was again central to Helen's progress and the success of the counselling.

Reflection on Helen's story

Helen shared her story in detail with the counsellor. For the first time in two years, she felt safe enough to disclose her feelings of guilt and shame. Helen had been struggling a great deal with these feelings, and her mood had gradually worsened. The counsellor gently encouraged her to explore and express these feelings. Helen did not feel judged, and was relieved to be able to share her concerns. The counsellor normalized the feelings, and began some mindfulness work with Helen. She also explained the process of acceptance and shared some acceptance and defusion techniques to enable Helen to gain a sense of being able to manage the feelings.

Helen's thinking was also explored, and the counsellor picked up on her expectation that she 'should not have been grumpy' with her husband. This was gently challenged, and Helen was taught to let go of the word 'should'. Helen was asked to step back and look at what occurred in her husband's final months. She was able to see that it was very demanding caring for her husband full-time, and she recalled often being very tired and grumpy as a result. Helen's tiredness and irritability were normalized, and unrealistic expectations of herself gradually challenged.

Helen felt the load of guilt and shame lightening. She learnt to treat herself with more kindness, and her mood lifted as a result.

LLCC TIPS: OVERCOMING GUILT AND SHAME

- Be aware of shame or guilt, and that they are normal emotions.
- Express these motions via talking or expressive activities such as art.
- There are links between thoughts, feelings of shame and guilt, and behaviours.
- Be aware of unhelpful thinking patterns, and practise challenging or reframing thoughts.

- Identify any unhelpful behaviours such as overeating, excessive alcohol or other self-harming behaviours, which may be being used to numb the shame or guilt.
- Practise mindfulness, and utilize ACT processes such as acceptance and defusion. The 'acceptance tool kit' described earlier is also useful with shame and guilt.
- Focus on strengths which can be used to deal with any issues that need attention.
- Narrative questioning can be useful as part of the conversation about guilt and shame.
- Work on self-belief.

Resources

Books

Brown, B. 2010, *The Gifts of Imperfection: Let go of who you think you're supposed to be and embrace who you are*, Hazelden Publishing, Minnesota.

Brown, B. 2012, *Daring Greatly: How the courage to be vulnerable transforms the way we live, love, parent, and lead*, Penguin, New York.

Edelman, S. 2013, *Change Your Thinking: Positive and practical ways to overcome stress, negative emotions and self-defeating behaviour using CBT*, HarperCollins Publishers, Sydney.

Harris, R. 2007, *The Happiness Trap: Stop struggling, start living*, Exisle Publishing, New South Wales.

Websites

ACT and mindfulness: www.actmindfully.com.au

Beyondblue: www.beyondblue.org.au

Black Dog Institute: www.blackdoginstitute.org.au/public/research/ehealth.cfm

Brené Brown's work on guilt and shame (including blogs): www.brenebrown.com

Phone apps

Smiling Mind: www.smilingmind.com.au

Chapter 9
Navigating change and transition

The last three years have been like one endless workday without rest for me. Now it's over . . . my poor mother doesn't need me . . . nor the boys either.

How free you must feel?

No . . . only unspeakably empty . . . Nothing to live for now.

—**HENRIK IBSEN,** *A DOLL'S HOUSE*

Change and transition are universal experiences in life, and counsellors commonly work with individuals dealing with these experiences. This chapter will take you through relevant background theory and explore various therapeutic approaches and strategies you might find useful in your work. Counsellors can support individuals going through change and transition to adapt emotionally, thereby reducing distress. The next chapter, on managing loss and grief, follows on well from this one, as these can result from such changes in life.

As you read this chapter, reflect on Annie's story and consider what approaches and strategies might assist her.

Annie's story

Annie grew up in Sydney and practised as an accountant. She met Joe, and they married and had a son. Joe was completing theological studies and training, and when he became a minister they were assigned a parish in Melbourne. They moved cities and a few months later, Annie came for counselling because she was feeling very anxious. She said that she was struggling with being a mother and a minister's wife, and she talked about all of the demands being placed on her and having little support.

Background

Life is like riding a bicycle. To keep your balance you must keep moving.

—ALBERT EINSTEIN

During our lives, we experience change and role transition many times, such as going to school, moving into adolescence, moving in with a partner, getting a job, having children, divorce and retirement, to name a few. Change and role transition in life can be very stressful and involve an array of emotions, both 'positive and negative', and a sense of loss and grief. It can be hard to deal with uncertainty in life, especially as humans tend to like a sense of control and security.

Change is defined as an act or process through which something becomes different, while transition is the process or a period of changing from one state or condition to another.[1] There are many different types of transition, including:

- life stage transitions (e.g. parenthood, retirement, empty nest)
- situational transitions (e.g. promotion, graduation, migration)
- gains (e.g. new house, financial windfall)
- relationship transitions (e.g. divorce, becoming a step-parent)
- illness-related transitions (e.g. chronic illness diagnosis)
- event-related transitions (e.g. PTSD, refugee status).

LLCC TIP
To understand the impact of transitions, consider one time of transition in your own life and reflect on what was involved, what the challenges were, how you felt, and how you moved through this time and mastered the transition.

LLCC management

Hearing the person's story and making sense of distress in terms of change and role transition is very important. The formulation process is very helpful in relation to change and transition (see Chapter 2). Review the top half of Figure 10, the formulation for Annie's story, which names the factors influencing Annie's distress; placing it in the context of change and role transition (and potentially loss and grief) proved to be very powerful for Annie. It relieved her fear that she was 'losing it' and made it very apparent that she had been through a lot and was under a lot of stress at the time.

A range of approaches and strategies can assist individuals with change and transition. These are detailed below.

- **Psycho-education** about change and its effects, and about times of transition in life can assist. It is important to explain to the person that change and transition can be very stressful and result in anxiety.
- **Expressing** thoughts and feelings associated with change and transition is vital. This may be through talking with family members, colleagues or a counsellor, or through expressive techniques such as art or music.
- It is helpful to establish or review personal **goals**, and consider how the change might assist in achieving the goals. Consider again the reasons for making a change, as well as the advantages and disadvantages of the change.[2]
- Sprague spoke of the importance of finding some **structure** to the day and week, continuing with activities of living, and over time reassessing the situation.[3]

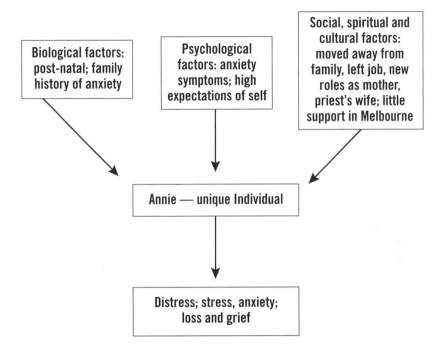

Figure 10: Formulation for Annie

Cognitive Behaviour Therapy

Researchers have looked at the cognitive–emotional process involved in change, and found that it involves:

- an evaluation of whether the change is relevant to wellbeing and personal goals
- secondary thoughts related to congruence between goals and the change's goals, plus confidence in success of proposed change.[4]

CBT can assist in managing change and transition via:

- ensuring pleasant and relaxing activities are scheduled into the week, even though the client might be very busy as a result of the change
- stress management via lifestyle measures and relaxation techniques
- problem-solving issues which arise as part of the change or transition
- being aware of unhelpful thinking patterns such as black-and-white thinking or catastrophizing, which might impact on levels of anxiety and mood, and working on more helpful thinking
- being aware of underlying beliefs that might influence thoughts and feelings at time of change — these might include, 'I should always be in

control' or 'Bad things should not happen to me' and how these might get in the way of adapting to new situations.

Acceptance and Commitment Therapy

The aim of ACT processes is to build more psychological flexibility to aid adaption to the change and new roles. ACT reminds us to focus on what is important in life. It can be helpful to encourage the client undergoing a lot of change to remind themselves of what they value, and to maintain focus on this throughout the change. Ensuring goals are in line with values is vital, and these measures will help the client find meaning in the process of change or transition.

Practising mindfulness can also assist the client to manage stress and not get caught up with worries about the future. Acceptance is an important process to discuss, as change is part of life and will be challenging at times. Defusion techniques assist with managing uncomfortable feelings which might arise (see p. 106).

Interpersonal Therapy

IPT identifies role transition as one of its key problem areas. We undergo many role transitions in life. Sometimes these bring joy, and sometimes distress. Exploring the range of feelings generated is helpful, as is normalizing the feelings. The IPT **timeline** is useful in demonstrating how symptoms of distress might relate to times of change or transition in life. This can raise awareness of the links for the client (see Annie's timeline).

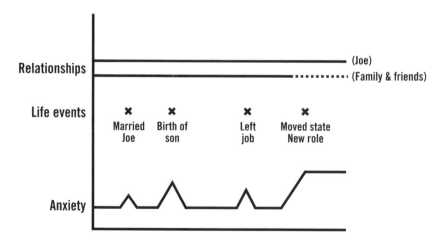

Figure 11: Annie's timeline

IPT highlights as a problem area the **loss and grief** that can stem from role transition. Role transitions are assisted through facilitating the expression of emotion and the grieving process. The principles of grief counselling covered in Chapter 9 can be applied. Acceptance of the loss of the old role is worked on. The positive and negative aspects of the old role can be explored, along with what has changed. It can be helpful to assist the client to consider the new role more positively, by asking about the positive aspects of the role and potential benefits. Enhancing social skills involved in the new role, along with self-belief, may be helpful. This may involve role-playing situations involved in the new role or exploring assertiveness. Exploring new social supports can also assist.

Narrative Therapy

Many aspects of Narrative Therapy can assist with adaption to change and role transition. Hearing the person's story fully, listening to their joys and fears, challenges and successes, is the foundation of narrative. The metaphor of a journey is often used to describe change and transition and is very appropriate. Relaying this to the client can assist, as well as drawing on their strengths to help them navigate the journey.

The narrative technique known as **migration of identity** is very powerful.[5] It was developed in relation to women experiencing domestic violence, who separate and go through a series of phases in the process of reincorporating their own identity into their lives. The metaphor has also been applied to migration and has been used in counselling work with refugees.[6] It has been applied to overcoming problematic behaviours such as addictions, and I would suggest that it is also applicable to a range of significant or challenging transitions in life. It involves three phases:

- life before the point of separation
- the 'liminal' stage, characterized by a condition of ambiguity, confusion and disorientation
- the reincorporation stage.[7]

These phases can be charted, with the three stages on the horizontal axis plotted against degrees of a sense of despair or a sense of wellbeing on the vertical axis. This chart can be used to map the separation from familiar life to the new life. The migration of identity map charts the difficult journey that clients can go through, and shows why they might remain still in some places or backtrack at other times. The counsellor may need to remind the person that even when people go back, this does not mean they are back at the very beginning. The migration of identity map shows that the overall journey is forwards and upwards.

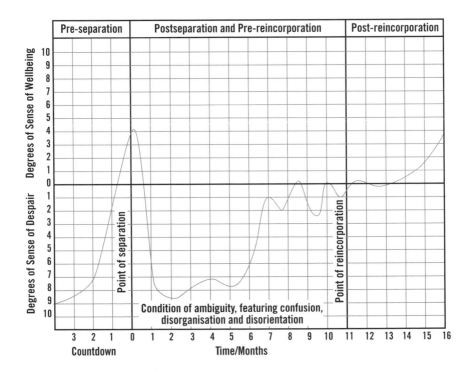

Figure 12: The migration of identity map[8]

LLCC TIP
A simple figure can also be drawn for clients, to illustrate the concept of moving forward despite setbacks. Draw a series of hills with a stick figure traversing them. Even though there will be dips in their travel, the direction in which the figure moves is still forwards.

Expressive therapies

Expressive therapies can foster self-awareness and insight in relation to change and transition. Writing a journal can be powerful as a record of the period of change, and to express feelings and set new goals. Art Therapy can provide as safe way to explore and express feelings, and can lead to new understanding. Examples of exercises include:

- the client drawing what is significant in their life at this time of change.
- the client drawing their feelings and keeping a journal of the drawings.
- the client drawing what brings them joy in life.[9]

Drawings can be done in session time and then discussed. The client is also likely to want to do some at home. Note that information from the unconscious mind might present itself in the drawings. Holding them up across the room from the client and asking them to describe their drawing often leads to a new perspective coming through; for example, something they hadn't thought of expressing might be seen in the drawing. Colours and styles used can also be reflected upon. For example, do they seem to reflect peace, turmoil, anger, sadness or joy?

Hypnotherapy

Hypnotherapy can assist through:

- reinforcement of **psycho-education** about change and transition
- **relaxation and self-hypnosis** for associated stress and anxiety
- **ego-strengthening** to build self-belief
- **direct suggestions** about using coping skills
- reinforcement of concepts and strategies from **CBT**, **ACT** and **IPT**.

Hypnotherapy may also utilize a **journey metaphor** to assist in coping with change or transition. Following is a script I have often used in this context. Notice it integrates concepts from other therapies, such as Narrative Therapy and Positive Therapy. Following this metaphor, the counsellor and client can discuss the client's experiences and reflections.

We are going to make a journey today. Imagine a path which leads into beautiful countryside. On this journey, you might see what is around you or hear sounds or feel yourself moving. As you follow the path, tap into your senses. There is a gentle breeze, the sunshine is pleasantly warm, and everything is green. As you walk along, you feel any tension in your body or mind disappearing. You can relax and enjoy the peace of nature.

The path leads down now towards a pond and stream. The water comes from higher up in the countryside, and it is fresh and clean. You can put your hand in and feel the temperature — you can even drink from it, or you might want to bathe your feet. There are some boulders near the pond to sit on, and you can relax for a while there. It is always important to rest from time to time on a journey.

You gather up some leaves and twigs and are mindful of their colours, the patterns on them, the feel of them, their textures. As a child, I wonder if you placed leaves and twigs into a stream and watched them float downstream? If you would like to, you can do this now. But first, there might be thoughts or feelings you would like to place on each leaf or twig. Maybe tiredness, fear or doubt. Spend a few moments doing this, then release the leaves and twigs into the stream. They will flow gently away, to a place where they need not be of concern.

It's time now to follow the path as it leads up a hillside. It is a gentle climb and there are a few steps in the path Gradually you notice that you can start to see out over trees. Up it goes until you reach a place near the top where there is a seat on which to sit and enjoy the view — you can see a long way from this place. And what a different perspective you have here compared with lower down. Sometimes a time of change can seem overwhelming but when we step back from it we can discover a different perspective: perhaps about the strengths we have used along the way; perhaps new meaning; maybe about how much we have grown along the way. I wonder which resources you have tapped into within yourself on your recent journey of change, and what wisdom you have acquired? Spend some time at this spot, breathing and reflecting.

And when you are ready, gradually follow the path back down, past the stream and bring yourself back to the here and now.

Positive Therapy

Positive Therapy focus on values and utilizing strengths, and is helpful in adapting to change and transition. Frederickson writes about the link between positive mood and adapting to stress, hence fostering positive emotions such as savouring and gratitude can assist in coping with change.[10] Tapping into creativity at times of change and transition is valuable, whether to relax or in relation to problem-solving. The client can be encouraged to make use of coping mechanisms they have built and found helpful in the past, such as gaining support from family, talking with friends or making lists. Connecting with loved ones should be encouraged, along with self-care. Finding meaning in the change and new roles is helpful. Positive Therapy has a focus on building resilience skills and flourishing, and the aim is to use positive coping skills to adapt and flourish in new environments and roles.[11] Flexibility is important and being in the moment to react to whatever is needed. Adopting a 'wait and see' attitude is helpful at times.

In summary

Life is full of change, which can be exciting and challenging. It can involve gains as well as losses, and associated grief can add to distress. To manage change, individuals need to be patient and compassionate towards themselves, and practise acceptance and flexibility. Expressing the full array of feelings and drawing on their strengths and coping skills can assist. Change and transition can provide opportunities for self-awareness and growth.

Reflection on Annie's story

The counsellor heard Annie's story and was struck by how much change and role transition she had been through. The counsellor carried out a formulation and when taking Annie through it — which highlighted having a young child, moving cities, leaving family behind, leaving her job and taking on a new role (minister's wife) — it also became apparent to Annie that she had experienced a lot of change. The counsellor also framed some of the change as involving loss and grief, and encouraged Annie to talk about her feelings.

Psycho-education about anxiety relieved some of Annie's worry about her symptoms, and she was taught some relaxation and mindfulness techniques to help with the anxiety symptoms. The counsellor also focused on cognitive techniques, as she had become aware that Annie had very high expectations of herself. Annie was taught to be more compassionate towards herself, and to take some time out to enjoy her hobby, scrapbooking. Annie was open to using hypnotherapy, and all of these strategies could therefore be reinforced in hypnosis. Ego-strengthening suggestions were incorporated, and she enjoyed the change metaphor in particular.

LLCC TIPS: NAVIGATING CHANGE AND TRANSITION

- Use known strengths.
- Be mindful or values and meaning.
- Process the change and any associated grief — talk about it.
- Practise mindfulness.
- Be creative and flexible.
- Grow acceptance.
- Tap into a positive mindset — practise optimistic thinking.
- Foster positive emotions.
- Foster self-compassion.
- Practise self-care, including stress management.

Resources

Books

McKissock, D. and M. 2012, *Coping with Grief* (4th ed.), HarperCollins Publishers, Sydney.

Price, S., Price, C. and McKenry, P. 2010, *Families and Change: Coping with stressful events and transitions* (4th ed.), Sage Publications, USA.

Websites

Australian Psychological Society: www.psychology.org.au

General information on grief: www.grieflink.asn.au

Psychology Today blog: www.psychologytoday.com

The American Psychological Association: www.apa.org (search for 'Change')

Phone apps

Breathe2Relax: http://t2health.dcoe.mil/apps/breathe2relax

Breathing Zone: www.breathing-zone.com

Meditation Oasis: http://www.meditationoasis.com/apps/

Smiling Mind: www.smilingmind.com.au

Chapter 10
Loss and grief counselling

Grief can be the garden of compassion. If you keep your heart open through everything, your pain can become your greatest ally in your life's search for love and wisdom.

—RUMI

Loss and grief are very common issues in the counselling setting. Individuals may come in seeking help because they are struggling with a recent loss or because of their sense of grief, or they might present with other concerns such as sleep problems, low mood or relationship issues. However, when you hear their story it often becomes apparent that they have experienced significant loss and grief, which is contributing to their concerns. An individual can experience loss that is death-related or non-death-related, including divorce, loss of one's job or ill health.

Here is the story of a young couple and their baby. As you read this case study, reflect on how you would support them and which approaches and strategies may assist.

David and Julie's story

David and Julie came to counselling together and sat holding hands. Three months previously they had been excited to be going to hospital for the birth of their first baby. Hours later Julie delivered their little girl, who was stillborn.

They were understandably devastated. They were able to spend time with their daughter, name her and dress her. There had been a funeral. They were supporting each other in coping with their loss, and their family was being very helpful. A friend suggested counselling might be another support.

Background

It is important to have a sound knowledge of the issues involved with loss and grief, so this chapter provides background information to understand these issues and to be able to provide appropriate management, including psycho-education, for clients. Remember that individuals will be unique in their responses, but there are some common threads to be aware of.[1]

First, some definitions:

- **Loss** involves separation from something that has meaning to us and to which we feel connected.
- **Grief** is the response to loss, and affects many aspects of the individual including their physical, emotional, behavioural, cognitive, social and spiritual self. It involves adaptation to the loss, and as loss often threatens our beliefs about the world, it takes time to re-adjust.[2]

Loss may occur suddenly or gradually, such as adapting to chronic illness. Individuals may hide loss, particularly if there is stigma or shame involved. There can be differences between men and women in grieving, or cultural differences, and individuals might not seek help with their grief because of these factors. Adjusting to loss takes time and effort; working with a counsellor can assist greatly.

There are numerous types of losses in life. Loss may involve death of a loved one or pet. It might be related to relationship breakdown, occupational losses, finances or ill health. Mobility or independence can be lost after an accident or illness. Refugees can experience multiple losses, including their homeland, belongings and family. A feeling of safety might be lost after a trauma such as rape.

In general, losses can be categorized as:

- **death or non-death** related

- **anticipated** loss, such as in terminal illness or divorce
- **disenfranchised** loss, that is, 'the grief that persons experience when they incur a loss that is not or cannot be openly acknowledged, publicly mourned, or socially supported'; examples are a parent grieving the loss of a child who suicides, or the potential loss of grandchildren when a child tells a parent they are in a same-sex relationship[3]
- **ambiguous** loss, that is, there is lack of clarity or certainty, such as a missing relative or changes in a partner's personality following a head injury or with dementia[4]
- **non-finite** loss, which refers to loss that occurs gradually over the lifespan, such as disability, dementia or infertility. 'Chronic sorrow' refers to those who are experiencing or caring for someone with a chronic or life-limiting condition resulting in disability.[5]

Loss can also be categorized as:

- **major or minor**, where major loss refers to death of a family member or involvement in a major trauma; remember, however, that minor losses, such as loss of the ability to drive, can still have a significant effect on the individual
- **primary or secondary**; an example of a primary loss is cancer, and related secondary losses could include loss of a body part or loss of the ability to work
- **internal versus external**; external losses can challenge internal ways of thinking about appearance, body image or gender and lead to grief reactions
- **chosen or imposed**; loss can result from our own choices, such as choosing to move countries, or it can be imposed, for example, fleeing a country due to persecution
- **direct versus indirect**; loss can occur through the experience of another person; for example, a parent can experience a loss that is affecting their child.[6]

There are a number of factors that influence our experience of grief. These include:

- previous life experience
- religious and philosophical backgrounds — spiritual beliefs can be protective
- behaviour modelled in family of origin
- gender — men and women may express or process grief in different ways; as a generalization, males through action and females through talking and expressing emotions

- current mental and physical health status
- biological; for example, a history of past depression or trauma
- the individual's available supports.

Grief is experienced in a number of ways, namely through feelings, physical sensations, cognitions and behaviours.[7]

Feelings can include shock, numbness, sadness, anger, guilt, anxiety, loneliness, helplessness, yearning, despair, depression and relief. Some of these can be more difficult to work through or manage, such as anger directed at others or anxiety which triggers an Anxiety Disorder.

Physical reactions include fatigue, breathing difficulties, muscle weakness, oversensitivity to noise or a sense of depersonalization.[8]

Cognitive reactions include disbelief, confusion, reduced memory and concentration, a sense of hopelessness or unreality, preoccupation with thoughts of the deceased, sense of presence and hallucinations.[9] Preoccupation with thoughts, images and memories of a deceased loved one is normal.

Behavioural reactions include crying, agitation, social withdrawal, sleep disturbances, appetite changes, absent-minded behaviour, searching and calling out, avoiding reminders of the deceased, restless overactivity, visiting places or carrying objects that remind one of the deceased.[10]

Grief is experienced in a number of ways, through feelings, physical sensations, cognitions and behaviours.

THE GRIEF PROCESS

Working through loss and the grief reaction takes time, and this is referred to as **the grief process**. There have been many theories about the grief process and some are described here.

- Grief involves adaptation to the loss. Loss and grief threaten our assumptions about the world and it takes time to readjust.[11]
- **Attachment** between individuals develops to maintain a state of balance in life, and loss and grief disturbs this balance. There can be a rollercoaster of emotions, from sadness to numbness, anger, guilt or anxiety.
- Bowlby's four stages model highlights numbness, preoccupation or yearning to recover the lost person, disorganization and despair, and

re-organisation.[12] Sanders described five phases of mourning: shock, awareness of loss, conservation–withdrawal, healing and renewal.[13]

- Note that the phase view of the grief process has been widely criticized as it implies that grieving is passive. Those opposed to the phase models, such as Attig, suggest that grief and mourning is an active process through which the griever relearns their world and how to live in it without the deceased.[14]

Grief involves adaptation to the loss and this take time.

Between 10 and 20 per cent of those grieving will experience **complicated or prolonged grief**, characterized by ongoing, problematic grief.[15] Many of the symptoms experienced in normal grief overlap with symptoms of depression, such as sadness, crying, loss of appetite, disturbed sleep and poor concentration. However, these symptoms gradually lessen over time. On some occasions, a depressive illness or an anxiety disorder may develop or, where there has been trauma, Post-traumatic Stress Disorder.

Factors that can complicate grief include:
- uncertain death or loss (e.g. missing persons)
- several losses at the one time
- poor quality of the lost relationship (ambivalent, hostile, dependent)
- self-blame, guilt
- past history of depression
- personality factors (dependent, narcissistic)
- unresolved previous losses
- past history of trauma such as child abuse
- attachment issues (insecure)
- social problems
- prolonged duration of grief
- repressed emotion
- death of a child
- sudden, unexpected death or loss
- long illness prior to death
- belief the loss was avoidable.[16]

Be mindful, too, that **anniversary reactions** can occur in relation to loss and grief. These include the anniversary of the death, the birthday of deceased,

Mother's or Father's Day, Christmas or other religious times of the year. At these times, the sense of loss and grief can reappear and can seem quite out of the blue for the client.

LLCC TIP

Discuss anniversary reactions with clients. Being prepared and understanding them can assist.

LLCC management

The management of loss and grief has been influenced by a number of people and theories. Understanding a client's losses and grief can guide the counsellor to the most appropriate and comprehensive management that can be provided. A few of the major theories informing loss and grief counseling follow.

Weenolsen devised a framework of **five levels of loss**:

- the primary level of loss, which tends to dominate an individual's perception of a 'loss' situation
- the secondary level/s of loss
- the holistic level of loss, involving the abstract losses associated with the primary and secondary losses; for example, a child's illness signifying loss of future hopes and dreams
- the self-conceptual level of loss, that is, the primary loss leads to changes in how the client sees themselves; part of the self might be perceived as loss, for example, an illness might lead the client to seeing themselves as 'sick' or 'less competent' or a burden on the family.
- the metaphorical level of loss, that is, the individual meaning a loss has when the client's beliefs are challenged.[17]

Worden devised **four tasks of mourning**. These are to accept the reality of the loss; to work through the pain of grief; to adjust to an environment without the lost person/object; and to emotionally relocate the lost person/object and move on with life.

- Accepting the reality of the loss occurs in steps. Initially there is numbness, shock and denial (seen as a defence mechanism to protect the individual from anxiety). Denial allows the person to face smaller parts of the experience rather than being overwhelmed by the entire thing. Both intellectual and emotional acceptance of the loss must take place. The reality of the situation might keep changing as the gravity of the loss unfolds, and will be revisited.

- Working through the pain of grief (sadness, loneliness, depressive feelings) takes time. The distress can be intense and attempts to avoid it may occur (stopping painful thoughts, distracting oneself by keeping busy, numbing through the use of alcohol).
- To adjust to an environment in which the lost person/object is missing, various adjustments are needed: external, internal and spiritual. External adjustments refers to functional changes, such as learning new skills and taking on new roles (e.g. managing finances) after the death of a loved one. These processes can be emotionally challenging and require internal adjustments. The person's spirituality might also be challenged or deepened through loss and grief.
- Worden also speaks of relocating the lost person and moving forward with life. This might involve maintaining a sense of connection with the lost person/object, and re-engaging with life.[18]

Worden noted that grievers need to 'act' in order to move through the grief process and the implication of his model is that mourning can be influenced by intervention from the outside, for example, through counselling.[19]

One of the most appealing grief management theories relates to **continuing bonds**. This theory is based on the fact that the client was connected to the deceased. It supports the client to continue the attachment with the person who has died. Continuing bonds involves exploring the meaning of the attachment, and encouraging the client to further develop their own identity after the loss. The deceased person might continue to be a role model after their death, they may represent certain values and the client might reflect on how their loved one would have guided them in certain situations (such as decision-making), or they might simply enjoy remembering them.[20]

Continuing bonds supports the client's continuing attachment to the person who has died.

US researcher and psychotherapist Robert Neimeyer has taken the continuing bonds theory forward. As grieving is viewed as a process of reconstructing a world of meaning that has been challenged by the loss, Neimeyer focuses on **meaning reconstruction** in grief therapy.[21] This involves the client telling their stories, and there may be a sense of their story being shattered by the grief. Retelling the story (literally or metaphorically) can be restorative, in addition to reconstructing its meaning in the client's ongoing life. This involves integrating the significance of the loss and extending the story of the loved one's existence in life-affirming ways. **Journalling** can be used as part of this process.[22]

A further model is the **dual process model**, referring to the need to both grieve the losses and to restore functioning as part of the grief journey.[23] There tends to be oscillation between these two processes. Grieving the losses involves more traditional grief work, whereas the restoration-perspective focuses on the additional stressors associated with a major loss, such as undertaking new tasks, organizing one's life without the deceased person, constructing some (and possibly new) meaning out of one's world, and developing a new identity.[24]

Here are some initial guidelines on how to assist the person who is grieving.

- Listen and empathize (the BATHE technique may be helpful — see p. 45).
- Ask about feelings and accept the intensity of emotions.
- **Normalize** the range of feelings and experiences.[25]

Normalizing the range of emotions is very powerful, as is reassurance.

- Give reassurance and information about grief, including explaining the physical symptoms which can occur.
- Discuss issues such as the funeral or viewing the body.
- Ask about sleep, eating and self-care generally.
- Provide information about management options.

Part of the counselling process will be monitoring for **risk** of self-harm and suicide. Clients are more vulnerable in the period after loss of a loved one. Assess regularly, and encourage the client to seek additional assistance as appropriate.

LLCC TIP
Monitor the grieving client carefully for risk of self-harm.

Social work lecturer, Michael Bull, writes about the behaviours which emerge during the grief process, categorizing them as life-enhancing or life-depleting. The former includes crying, talking, accepting assistance, self-care and seeking out symbolic connection with the deceased. Life-depleting behaviours often occur as part of avoidance of distressing emotions and can involve substance use, high-risk taking behaviours, compulsive or excessive behaviours (shopping, working, gambling), social isolation, agitation, aggression, anxiety-driven behaviours and suicide attempts.[26] The counsellor can monitor these behaviours and guide the person towards life-enhancing behaviours. It is also important to monitor the client for complicated grief.

Worden described grief therapy as involving:

- understanding the process of grief, and realizing that it is normal to have positive as well as negative feelings about the lost person or object
- sharing thoughts and feelings about the loss and reviewing what it means to the individual

LLCC TIP

Ask the client to bring in some photos or mementos of the lost person or object, and look at them together. It can also be helpful for the person to create a folder or scrapbook of mementos about the lost person or object.

- identifying and expressing the full range of emotions associated with the loss, such as guilt or anger; one way to do this is to talk about things they miss or don't miss about the person
- **problem-solving** ways of coping with the troublesome feelings resulting from the loss, practical problems, or new ways of coping in life
- eventually moving forward, and recognizing that this does not mean giving up on the lost person or object, but rather 'finding an appropriate place' for them in our emotional lives.[27]

Cognitive Behaviour Therapy

The following aspects of CBT can be helpful at different stages of grieving:

- psycho-education about loss and grief and the CBT approach
- behavioural strategies such as **relaxation** to reduce stress and aid sleep
- problem-solving strategies
- being aware of unhelpful thinking patterns and learning to manage them (see the study regarding Helen on pp. 166 and 172)
- retelling the story of loss and grief may involve the client being exposed to distressing images or feelings; the counsellor must be able to create safety and stay with the person until the images or feelings can be experienced

with less distress[27]
- reviewing progress regularly, to assist the person to see that they are moving forwards.

Dr Sheila Clark, an Australian GP with a special interest in grief, developed **the grief map** to help clients see and celebrate their progress. The map also educates clients about the array of emotions they may be feeling and it can trigger useful discussion, such as about continuing bonds and finding meaning from the loss. A copy is included in the Appendix (see p. 301) and guidelines for use of the map include the following:
- Underline the mountains relevant to your journey, and cross out the ones which are not relevant.
- Are there additional mountains to include? If so, add them.
- If some mountains are especially big or difficult, then make them taller.
- Fill in each mountain to the height you feel you have climbed.
- Then look at the map and ask yourself, 'What issues have I dealt with? What successes can I identify? What issues do I still need to work on? Where do I need some help?'[29]

Acceptance and Commitment Therapy

ACT can assist with managing intrusive thoughts and uncomfortable feelings. Acceptance is central as loss and death are part of life, and they involve distressing emotions. Practising **mindfulness** is key, as it can help relieve stress, raise awareness of and assist with managing emotions. It is part of learning to sit with emotions (see the 'Being with an emotion' exercise, p. 106). Defusion techniques — such as placing a thought on a cloud and watching it float away, or putting thoughts on leaves and letting them float downstream — can also assist.

Interpersonal Therapy

IPT identifies loss and grief as a key area to work on. The counsellor relates the timing of the loss or grief to the onset of symptoms of distress, explores the client's relationship with the lost person or object, is supportive and empathetic in exploring the client's feelings associated with the loss and links the feelings to the loss. They help the client to communicate the loss and to garner support from existing networks or create new ones. Grief resolves and new attachments are fostered.

Ask the client to consider what they have learnt through the loss. Have they grown in any way, developed strengths or discovered true friends?

Reviewing progress can be a powerful tool in recovering from a loss. Ask the client if they could have coped as well 3 or 6 months ago, for example. What resources have they found within themself that have helped them cope?

Narrative Therapy

Narrative Therapy involves hearing the client's story and focuses on the person's strengths and resources throughout the story, and in managing the grief. Many grievers wish to stay connected to their loved one but might believe they are meant to be saying goodbye to them. Narrative Therapy encourages the client to 'say hello again' to the person they are grieving. This involves incorporating into the present what has been lost, for example, holding on to the influence (or some other meaningful aspect) of that person.[30] By 'saying hello again' to their loved one, the client can have an ongoing connection with the deceased while still learning to live a life without them physically present.[31] This is consistent with 'continuing bonds' (see p. 191) and the dual process model (see p. 192).

The 'saying hello again' metaphor involves asking the client questions along the lines of:

- 'If you were seeing yourself through [deceased's name] eyes now, what would you be noticing about yourself that you could appreciate?'
- 'What difference would it make to how you feel if you were appreciating this in yourself right now?'
- 'What would [deceased's name] have said or done in certain situations?'
- 'Can you see their characteristics in your sibling or child?'

An example of the value of 'saying hello again' is shown in the following case study.

Nicola's story

Nicola was twenty years old when she came to counselling. Her father had died suddenly 12 months previously, and her mother was concerned about Nicola's mood. Nicola shared the story of her life and her father. They had been very close and had done a lot of sailing together, and he had always been there at her sporting events during school years. Nicola was struggling with the loss. She missed him terribly.

In the first sessions, the focus was on connecting with Nicola, hearing her story and assessing mood and risk. She was struggling with low mood and disturbed sleep. The counsellor encouraged her to address her lifestyle, including exercise, and to use relaxation to aid sleep.

The concept of 'saying hello again' was introduced. A strong memory of him was his big hands, especially when they were sailing, and they made her feel safe. But Nicola kept coming back to the belief that he was gone.

Two interventions assisted Nicola and created a shift in her mood and thinking. Firstly, the counsellor had been close to her own father, and he had died several year before. Although not the same situation, some self-disclosure was powerful. Nicola's eyes opened and she commented that perhaps the counsellor could understand.

Also, at that time the counsellor had a young son and had noted that at times her son had mannerisms and facial expressions similar to her own father. The connection was made that although Nicola's father had died, his influence lived on in her genetics and any children she might have in the future.

These interventions marked a significant improvement in Nicola's wellbeing.

Hypnotherapy

Hypnotherapy can assist with:

- psycho-education about loss and grief
- normalizing feelings
- relaxation and self-hypnosis
- direct suggestions about self-care
- ego-strengthening suggestions about progress, strengths and resources
- indirect suggestions through metaphor, such as adapting the journey script (see p. 181) to a grief journey.
- reinforcing problem-solving
- expressing related emotions
- attending to any unfinished business through talking with the deceased, via a hypnotic technique involving regression to just before the time of their death; sound training in hypnotherapy is required for this technique, and care must be taken when trauma has been involved.

Expressive therapies

Art Therapy can assist with expressing the emotions involved in grief, as can journalling. Sometimes there are still things that need to be said to the deceased, and it can help to say these out loud at the graveside, or in a poem or letter. Another useful technique for grief is the **memory box**. The box (any box or container can be used) can be decorated with various materials. The client places into the box various items which trigger positive memories of the person who has died. These may include photographs, special cards or small belongings. They can bring out the box whenever they want to connect with the loved one.[32]

Rituals can also assist with the processing of emotions. Funerals are an example of a ritual in society to help the bereaved. In the same way, very simple psychological rituals can help us to release emotions which might have been back holding the client's progress. Rituals focus on letting go of troublesome emotions and mark a time for change and a new beginning.[33]

LLCC TIP
Only consider a ritual if you feel the client is emotionally ready.

Here are some important guidelines for planning a ritual:

- Think about the theme of the ritual, and decide on the goal.
- Take time to plan the ritual carefully.
- Keep it simple.
- Incorporate elements or symbols that are meaningful to the client.
- Are there things they particularly want to say or express?
- Do they want to have music?
- Choose the right time and place — indoors or outdoors?
- How does the client want to feel at the end of the ritual? What do they want to be different?
- Always end the ritual with something positive.
- Take time to reflect afterwards.

Here is an example of a ritual. A young woman, improving after having had some mental health problems, wants to let go of the remaining guilt and grief. She also wants to celebrate her improvement and what she has learnt about herself. She decides to buy some helium-filled balloons and plans for each one to represent something different. One will represent guilt and another grief. She chooses the brightest coloured balloons to represent her hard work in recovery, and the positive things about herself: her strength and courage. The young woman makes a cake and has a special celebration. She lets go of the balloons representing guilt and grief. The brightly coloured balloons representing positive things become the centrepiece at her table and she shares the celebration with her family and best friend.

Positive Therapy

In loss and grief Positive Therapy may incorporate:

- identifying the client's strengths and resources, and encouraging greater use of them
- fostering positive emotions, including gratitude and kindness
- encouraging the client to engage in life, including leisure and creative activities
- fostering social support and connection
- mindfulness, self-care and positive coping skills
- focusing on values and purpose, meaning and hope.

Bibliotherapy and e-mental health

There are a number of helpful books. A good starting point is *Coping With Grief* by Dianne McKissock and Mal McKissock. *After Suicide: Help for the bereaved* by Dr Sheila Clark is also excellent. The websites listed in 'Resources' further provide valuable information that can be helpful in terms of education and tapping into community resources.

In summary

Loss and grief are part of life, and grief can be experienced in a number of ways, including an array of feelings, physical sensations, cognitions and behaviours. Working through the grief process takes time and involves adaptation to the loss. This is because of the role of attachment to the lost person or object. The 'continuing bonds' theory supports continuing this attachment with a person who has died. Continuing bonds also involves exploring the meaning of the attachment, and encouraging the client to further develop their own identity after the loss. This fits with the 'dual process model', referring to the need to both grieve the losses and to restore functioning as part of the grief journey. There are many useful approaches and techniques to assist the client working through loss and grief. These include hearing the story, the grief map, 'saying hello again' and expressive techniques.

Reflection on David and Julie's story

David and Julia shared their story and cried. They were devastated by the loss of their daughter, but also certain that she would play an important part in their ongoing lives. David was working on a cubby house in the backyard, and Julie had been making a memory box with mementos of their daughter. Julie would talk regularly with family and friends about her loss and grief, but David was more reluctant.

They were concerned for each other and supportive, but struggling to understand the differences between them in how they were managing their grief. Providing information about grief, and normalizing not only their experiences but expression of their grief was helpful. The differences between men and women was touched on. They were able to share with each other how they felt and what their different actions meant to them. They continued to move forward with their grief, with their daughter part of their lives.

LLCC TIPS: MANAGING LOSS AND GRIEF

Suggestions for the client to help manage their grief include the following.

■ Allow grief time each day — say 15 to 20 minutes — in which to talk or journal about the loss, or to have a cry.

■ Attend to self-care, including relaxation, walking in nature or pampering. Consider whether time off work is needed.

■ Name the problems, which can then be problem-solved. Note, however, that it is important to not make any major decisions in the first 12 months.

■ Identify the losses and link mood with the loss.

■ Continue existing relationships and seek support.

■ Use spiritual support if meaningful.

■ Explore and express emotions.

■ Get some advice on dealing with practical issues or managing anniversaries.

■ Practise self-compassion.[34]

Resources

Books

Clark S. 1995, *After Suicide: Help for the bereaved*, Hill of Content, Melbourne.

McKissock, D. and M. 2012, *Coping with Grief* (4th ed.), HarperCollins, Sydney.

McKissock, D. and M. 2003, *Bereavement Counselling: Guidelines for practitioners*, Bereavement Care Centre, New South Wales.

Neimeyer, R. (ed.) 2001, *Meaning, Reconstruction and the Experiences of Loss*, American Psychological Association, Washington.

Neimeyer, R. (ed.) 2012, *Techniques of Grief Therapy: Creative practices for counseling the bereaved*, Routledge, New York.

White, C. and Denborough, D. (eds) 1998, *Introducing Narrative Therapy: A collection of practice-based writings*, Dulwich Centre Publications, Adelaide.

Websites

Australian Centre for Grief and Bereavement, 'Resources': www.grief.org.au/
resources

Australian Psychological Society: www.psychology.org.au

Bereavement Care Centre: www.bereavementcare.com.au/resources/books

Open Leaves Books: www.openleaves.com.au/categories/Loss-and-Grief/Grief-
Counselling/

GriefLink, general information: www.grieflink.asn.au

NHS, stories, articles, advice and support: www.nhs.uk/LiveWell/bereavement/
Pages/bereavement.aspx

NHS, suicide and other sudden, traumatic death: www.nhs.uk/Livewell/
Suicide/Documents/Help%20is%20at%20Hand.pdf

US National Library of Medicine, Medline Plus for information regarding
bereavement and related issues, specific conditions, research and resources for
counsellors and clients: www.nlm.nih.gov/medlineplus/bereavement.html

US National Library of Medicine, MedLine Plus grief fact sheet: https://www.
nlm.nih.gov/medlineplus/ency/article/001530.htm

Phone apps

Breathe2Relax: http://t2health.dcoe.mil/apps/breathe2relax

Breathing Zone: www.breathing-zone.com

Meditation Oasis: http://www.meditationoasis.com/apps/

PTSD Coach Australia: http://at-ease.dva.gov.au/veterans/resources/mobile-
apps/ptsd-coach/

Smiling Mind: www.smilingmind.com.au

Chapter 11
A trauma-informed approach

I am not what happened to me, I am what I choose to become.

—CARL JUNG

Many clients will have experienced trauma/s of some kind during their lives. Examples include domestic violence, childhood physical or sexual abuse, emotional trauma, accidents such as motor vehicle or workplace accidents, or trauma related to natural disasters, violent crimes or some medical procedures. Refugees may have experienced significant trauma, and members of the defence forces or emergency services are often exposed to trauma. Trauma can have significant short- or long-term impacts on the individual, and can involve a great deal of loss and grief. Some individuals will have a severe and persisting reaction to trauma and will need specialized assistance.

This section provides an introduction to this area of counselling, with the aim of increasing understanding of the area and developing an approach to assist clients who have experienced trauma. Further study or training may be required to feel confident in managing clients who have experienced trauma. To begin, read Josie's story and reflect on her experience as you work through this section.

Josie's story

Josie and her husband decided to take a holiday. While on a day trip to a tourist centre, they heard gunfire. They ran for their lives, and with other tourists they took cover. Eventually the gunman was caught and they were safe. A number of lives had been lost.

Josie saw the counsellor soon after returning home, feeling very anxious.

Background

A traumatic event is one in which an individual experiences, witnesses or is confronted with actual or serious injury or threatened death. In a number of Western countries, approximately 75 per cent of individuals have been found to have experienced a traumatic event at some point in their lives, and most will experience more than one.[1,2] There can be single-incident trauma, repeated trauma and developmental trauma (such as neglect). Also, historical trauma can result from massive group trauma such as experienced in war, and intergenerational trauma from the psychological effects experienced by people who live with those impacted by trauma.[3]

Reactions to trauma will vary from person to person. A range of reactions occur, from shock and acute distress, to numbness and disconnection. Memory of the events can be affected. There can be an impact on the client's sense of safety and self-efficacy. Physical health can also be impacted, with greater susceptibility to illness and pain.[4] The acute reactions often settle, but when severe anxiety symptoms occur within one month of exposure to extreme traumatic stressor, it is called an Acute Stress Disorder.

Some clients may go on to develop Major Depression or Post-traumatic Stress Disorder (PTSD). PTSD can occur after they or someone close to them is exposed to threatened serious injury or death. The client may experience continued intrusive symptoms (images, dreams, flashback, distress), persistent emotions such as fear, anger, guilt, depression, persistent hyper-alertness, problems with sleep or memory/concentration, and they might avoid any reminders of the trauma and experience feeling dissociated from self or surroundings. Symptoms can persist for more than a month, and daily functioning may be impacted. Remember, too, that some people will develop PTSD at a much later time.[5]

LLCC management

Help or do not harm the patient.

—THOMAS INMAN

It is vital to be on the alert for a history of trauma exposure when hearing client's stories, and to enquire sensitively about trauma during the assessment process. It is also important not to assume that if the client is presenting with the effects of one trauma, they have not been exposed to other traumas. It can be very difficult for clients to raise or discuss trauma, as it is difficult to revisit memories associated with uncomfortable feelings, and there can be a range of emotions attached to trauma including anxiety, shame and guilt.

Researchers Briere and Scott have devised general guidelines for assessment of trauma exposure. The aim is to assist the client, and to ensure that they are not re-traumatized. At the outset, it is essential that rapport and trust are established between the client and counsellor. The counsellor will also need to gauge the client's capacity to manage discussion about the traumatic events. Discussion should only proceed if a client is assessed as having the stability to tolerate this and to remain safe. Otherwise the discussion should be delayed. In addition, counsellors might avoid the topic because of their own discomfort talking about it. Counsellors may need to work on their awareness of trauma and their own response to it. If engaging in discussion about trauma with clients, it is best for the counsellor to have a calm approach and manner.[6]

Other guidelines include the following:

- Describe traumatic events in behavioural terms, or using the words used by the client.
- Monitor the client carefully, so that the pace of discussion or direction can be changed if the client becomes anxious or unsettled.
- Respond to client disclosures and expressions of emotions in a way that demonstrates warmth, support and respect.
- Acknowledge their courage in discussing the trauma.
- Pace the discussion and sessions.
- Foster mutual learning (for both client and counsellor).
- Seek regular feedback from the client.
- Be open to referring clients to appropriate clinicians or agencies.

Briere and Scott also suggest some opening statements that can be used to open up discussions about trauma:

- 'If it is okay with you, I'd like to ask you some questions about your past. These are questions that I ask every client I see, so I can get a better sense of what he or she has been through.'

- 'I'd like to ask you some questions about experiences you may have had in the past. If you feel uncomfortable at any time, please let me know. Okay?'[7]

Remember that a comprehensive assessment is very important, including an assessment of mood, anxiety, risk of self-harm and suicide, as well as substance use. There is a range of assessment tools for trauma. An example of a screening tool for PTSD follows:

1. 'Have you had nightmares about the situation/trauma or thought about it when you did not want to?'

2. 'Have you tried hard not to think about it, or gone out of your way to avoid situations that reminded you of it?'

3. 'Do you feel you are constantly on guard, watchful or easily startled?'

4. 'Do you feel numb or detached from others, from activities or from your surroundings?'

If the client answers yes to two or more of these questions, a diagnosis of PTSD is probable.[8] Further tools can be found at www.phoenixaustralia.org

Trauma-informed practice

The general approach used in the mental health area when working with trauma is **trauma-informed practice**. This approach recognizes the prevalence of trauma and is sensitive to the impacts of trauma on the wellbeing of individuals and communities.[9] It aims to engage the client, and to make links between trauma and mental health or substance use issues. It requires having competence in relation to gender and culture.[10]

Trauma-informed models of care and guidelines have been developed in many settings across the world, and with different populations of clients. The underlying principles of this practice include:

1. **Trauma awareness**: having an understanding of trauma and how it impacts individuals.

2. **Emphasis on safety**: building physical, emotional and cultural safety for clients and counsellors that reduces exposure to triggers for re-traumatization.

3. Opportunities for **choice, collaboration and connection**: developing circumstances that foster choice, personal control, predictability and empowerment.

4. **Strengths-based and skill building**: identifying and utilizing strengths to develop coping skills that promote resilience and hopefulness.[11]

In using the trauma-informed approach, it is vital to be aware of and watch out for signs of the trauma response during counselling sessions. These can include sweating, breathing more quickly, muscle tension, a flood of strong emotions, shaking, staring into the distance or becoming disconnected from the conversation.[12] If this response occurs, pay careful attention to the client, offer verbal support with reassuring statements, such as, 'It's all right to cry, just let the shaking happen, it will end on its own.' Remain present and continue to offer grounding and calming statements. Encourage self-efficacy and collaboration by asking, '*What do you need now to feel safe?*'[13]

LLCC TIP
A useful grounding technique when working with trauma involves asking the client:
- 'What are three things you can see?'
- 'What are three things you can hear?'
- 'What are three things you can touch?'
Asking these questions can be helpful for the client at the end of the session.

Psychological first aid may be needed in the first instance following trauma. This involves providing compassionate support, ensuring safety, providing comfort, stabilizing those affected who are overwhelmed with reassurance and containment or safety, gathering information to prioritize response, providing practical assistance, connecting the client with social supports, providing psycho-education and linking the client to appropriate services.[14]

Note that there are group programs for trauma, as well as individual therapy. All require consistency, education and healthy boundaries and expectations, for example: consider what can be done and not done; and back-up plans for the client when the counsellor is not at work (such as after-hours services or emergency contacts).[15]

A range of therapies is utilized in working with trauma, namely:
- trauma-focused CBT and Eye Movement Desensitisation and Reprocessing (EMDR) — note that these have a strong evidence base in trauma[16]

- MBCT and ACT
- Narrative Therapy
- Expressive therapies, and others.

Note that EMDR was developed by Francine Shapiro to reduce the distress of traumatic memories. With EMDR, the counsellor uses questioning to desenstitize the client through imaginal exposure to the traumatic memory. The client is directed to focus on associated thoughts, emotions and sensations, as they also focus on the counsellor's finger movements.[17] This therapy requires attendance at further training (see 'Resources' at the end of this chapter).

The LLCC approach incorporates **CBT**, **MBCT**, **ACT**, **Narrative Therapy**, **Hypnotherapy**, **Positive Therapy**, **Bibliotherapy and e-mental health**, and some aspects of **expressive therapies**. Experience and training are necessary to utilize these in trauma. An outline follows, and counsellors will need to gauge their level of skill and training in relation to working in this area.

Preliminary work may involve **Motivational Interviewing** and overcoming barriers to counselling. Establishing the client's priorities and hopes is important, as is setting management goals. **Psycho-education** about trauma is the foundation of many of the therapies, an example being about memory. It can be helpful to discuss how memories are formed, with positive or negative associations. For example, when a client has a panic attack in the car, the car becomes a place of fear, triggering anxiety. The laying down of memories involves different parts of the brain, and one system in the brain allocates emotion to an event and places it in a time sequence. However, during stressful events, the processing of memories can be interrupted and some clients will recall the trauma as a disturbing state (incorporating both emotions and senses). There can be particular memory problems in PTSD, including poor short-term memory, flashbacks or patchy recollection of the trauma

Trauma-focused CBT

An adaptation of CBT for trauma, **trauma-focused CBT** involves psycho-education, symptom management (such as strategies to manage anxiety symptoms), arousal reduction, **exposure** and cognitive restructuring (identifying unhelpful thoughts and beliefs, challenging them and developing more helpful alternatives). The theory is that exposure leads to habituation, or lessening of anxiety.[18] When exposure is used, an exposure hierarchy is established (see the spider example on p. 95).

Cognitive processing is another form of CBT which addresses key themes of safety, trust, power and control, self-esteem and intimacy. Underlying beliefs of incompetence and the world being a dangerous place are identified, and the focus is on cognitive restructuring through exploration, reevaluation and establishing new perspectives.[19]

Here is an example of the steps used in exposure for PTSD:

1. An initial exposure session is conducted, to help the client gain confidence in telling their story. This is done with eyes open, in the past tense, checking anxiety regularly by using scaling questions (0–10). The counsellor looks for parts of the story that are 'hot' or associated with emotion.

2. The next step is to retell the story in the present tense with eyes closed. The client is encouraged to stay with the memory and the anxiety level is monitored. This is repeated until the anxiety level goes down. Reassurance is provided.

3. If new information is accessed, this can be reflected back and thoughts around it explored. Again, scaling questions are used to monitor anxiety.

4. If a memory that is higher on the exposure scale intrudes, attempt to bring the client back to the original memory. If this is not possible, reassure the client and return to step 1.

Mindfulness-based Cognitive Therapy

MBCT is used in trauma and involves:

- learning relaxation to reduce arousal, and body-scanning methods to learn acceptance of sensations
- practising mindfulness of thoughts to foster acceptance of them
- exposure techniques to reduce avoidance, such as learning to sit with uncomfortable emotions while delaying unhelpful behaviours (such as consuming alcohol) via mindfulness meditation
- developing more compassionate thoughts about oneself.

Acceptance and Commitment Therapy

Equally, the key processes of ACT can be very helpful in trauma:

- mindfulness, or contact with the present moment — to reduce stress, and to notice feelings and thoughts
- defusion of feelings and thoughts — for example, 'Being with an emotion' (see p. 106), or defusing unhelpful thoughts
- acceptance of uncomfortable feelings, thoughts and suffering in life
- self-as-context — to notice thoughts and feelings without judging them or struggling with them
- values — focusing on what is important to the client
- committed action and effort.[20]

Interpersonal Therapy

IPT may be used as the key therapy, especially where relationships are being significantly impacted. The nature of the distress can be identified and a timeline can help link the distress with trauma. Any loss and grief triggered by the trauma can be explored. IPT is readily used in an integrated way with other therapies such as CBT.

Narrative Therapy

Narrative Therapy is very applicable to trauma. The process of sharing the story can be very powerful for the client. The language that is used is important — normalizing the person's response to abnormal events can assist, as can externalizing the problem. It can be very empowering to move from the dominant problem-saturated story of the impact of the trauma to an alternative story of resourcefulness and survival. New meaning may arise, and narrative questioning can assist with this process (see p. 111). Culture driven ideas may need to be explored, for example, that a woman who has been assaulted is somehow 'damaged'. Challenging this notion and placing the dominant story in the social context can lead to other possibilities becoming apparent.[22]

Hypnotherapy

Hypnosis can assist in trauma through helping with stress management and anxiety symptoms. Ego-strengthening and focusing on the client's coping skills and strengths, can be helpful. Establishing a safe place in the mind, and using an anchor is also particularly useful. Exposure in the imagination (imaginal), similar to the CBT technique outlined, above can be used and helpful cognitions can be reinforced. Techniques for expressing associated emotions, such as anger or guilt, can be used.

Positive Therapy

Aspects of Positive Therapy resonate with trauma-informed therapy, namely:
- identifying and utilizing strengths
- working with values
- encouraging social connection, especially supportive connections, such as supportive friends or family and peer support groups
- focusing on meaning
- emphasizing hope and resilience
- fostering self-compassion.

Expressive therapies

Expressive therapies can assist the client to express and work through emotions, in activities such as making a collage of the emotions. **Journalling** can be used to enable the person to work through the traumatic incidents, not only in writing about events but also through describing their emotional reactions. They might need to do this in steps. Journalling can help the client process the memories, ascribing emotions to particular events, and may also be integrated into CBT.

Bibliotherapy and e-mental health

Bibliotherapy and e-mental health can provide psycho-education and management strategies. Authors Bass and Davis have written a particularly useful book, *The Courage to Heal: A guide for women survivors of child sexual abuse.* This is a self-help book and there is also a workbook available. Further information is provided in 'Resources' at the end of this chapter.

In summary

Reactions to trauma will vary from person to person. Some clients might go on to develop Major Depression or PTSD. The general approach used when working with trauma is trauma-informed practice, which is sensitive to the impacts of trauma on the wellbeing of individuals and communities. A range of therapies are utilized in working with trauma, including Trauma-focused CBT and Eye Movement Desensitization and Reprocessing (EMDR), MBCT and ACT, Narrative Therapy, Hypnotherapy and expressive therapies. Further training may be required to work safely and effectively in this area.

Reflections on Josie's story

Josie was struggling with anxiety symptoms following the trauma she had experienced, and she was later diagnosed with PTSD. She did not feel safe in any environment where there was a crowd of people. The counsellor began by building a sense of safety in the counselling environment and in relation to Josie's home and working life. An assessment was done, and revealed that Josie had experienced anxiety and depression in the past and had used medication at that time.

Ways to manage anxiety were discussed and Josie started to engage in daily walks and listening to meditation CDs she had used in the past. She found it helpful to talk through the different emotions she was feeling, and as she began journalling these Josie found mindfulness an interesting concept and could see how being mindful could bring her back to the moment rather than ruminating on the traumatic events. Being able to sit with the different emotions and breathe into them was helpful.

Josie decided to again utilize medication to aid her recovery, and this helped her gradually carry out exposure to situations where there were crowds, such as buses and cafés, starting with times when there were just a few people, and gradually building up to busier times. Her confidence grew over time, and the effects of the trauma reduced.

LLCC TIP: DEALING WITH TRAUMA

- Recognize that it has been a very distressing experience and focus on feeling safe and secure.
- Avoid overusing alcohol or other drugs.
- Express feelings rather than bottling them up — through talking, writing or activities such as sport.
- Let key family and friends know what support is needed, whether practical or emotional.
- Maintain a normal routine and do activities usually enjoyed.
- Rest when able, and use relaxation techniques.
- Eat well and do some exercise.
- Problem-solve what needs to be done.
- Be aware that a recent trauma can stir up memories from past traumas, and focus on keeping these memories separate.
- Seek professional help if necessary.

Resources

Books

Bass, E. and Davis, L. 2008, *The Courage to Heal: A guide for women survivors of child sexual abuse* (20th anniversary ed.), Collins Living, New York.

Curran, L. 2013, *101 Trauma-informed Interventions: Activities, exercises and assignments to move the client and therapy forward*, PESI Publishing and Media, USA.

Curran, L. 2010, *Trauma Competency: A clinician's guide*, PESI Publishing and Media, USA.

Davis, L. 1990, *The Courage to Heal Workbook: A guide for women and men survivors of child sexual abuse*, HarperCollins, New York.

Ringel, S. and Brandell, J. 2012, *Trauma: Contemporary directions in Theory, Practice, and Research*, Sage Publications, Los Angeles.

Websites

Abuse, domestic violence and sexual assault, with links and articles: www.nhs.
uk/livewell/abuse/pages/violence-and-sexual-assault.aspx

American Psychological Society: www.apa.org/topics/trauma/index.aspx

'Coping with a disaster or traumatic event', Centers for Disease Control and
Prevention: www.bt.cdc.gov/mentalhealth/index.asp

EMDR training: www.emdr.com (this is the US website; check for related groups
in other countries, such as www.emdr.com.au for information about Australia
and New Zealand).

General information on trauma: www.beyondblue.org.au and www.psychology.
org.au

New Zealand mental health resources: www.mentalhealth.org.nz/get-help/a-z

Phoenix Australia Centre for Posttraumatic Mental Health: www.phoenixaustralia.
org

PTSD resource: www.nhs.uk/Conditions/Post-traumatic-stress-disorder/Pages/
Treatment.aspx

South African Depression and Anxiety Group: www.sadag.org/

Phone apps

Breathe2Relax: http://t2health.dcoe.mil/apps/breathe2relax

Breathing Zone: www.breathing-zone.com

Meditation Oasis: http://www.meditationoasis.com/apps/

Smiling Mind: www.smilingmind.com.au

Chapter 12
Working on relationship issues

Being deeply loved by someone gives you strength, while loving someone deeply gives you courage.

—LAO TZU

Humans are social beings, and relationship issues will often impact on the wellbeing of a client or couple who present for counselling. The importance of always exploring significant relationships with an individual client has been touched on previously in relation to the genogram and the interpersonal inventory (see p. 109). Along with taking background information, these tools lead to greater insight into the client's family and partner relationships, along with levels of support or conflict issues. In this chapter the focus will be on couple relationship issues, although many of the principles can apply to other relationships.

Chris and Leanne's story

Chris and Leanne have been partners for 10 years. They were both previously married and have several adult children. Chris runs his own business and Leanne is a property manager. They live in separate houses but spend a lot of time together and hope to cohabitate in the future.

Their main issue is their different styles in managing conflict. Chris grew up with a father who would explode with anger, while Leanne grew up in a family in which anger was expressed through lively conversation. Leanne also worries about the Chris's business. As a result there is tension in the relationship and they are having doubts about the future.

Background

I trained in couple therapy 20 years ago and have worked with many couples since then. The training I undertook adopted an integrative approach and spoke of the value of looking at couple work through various lenses. Feminist theory, attachment theory, Family Therapy, CBT and Narrative Therapy were explored, and as part of the training we worked with clients in teams, with one person counselling and the remainder acting as a reflective team. My work with couples has continued to be integrative, because although there may be common issues, no two couples are the same.

Relationships are central to life. They can bring great joy, but also great stress. When there are significant problems in partner relationships, the client's mental and physical health can be affected. They may experience more illness, from mild illness to severe physical health issues. Mental health issues can also be triggered, including anxiety and depression, substance use issues and self-harming behaviours. In addition, the counsellor must always be aware of the potential for **domestic violence** in relationships. As a result, being alert for these issues and doing a thorough assessment is vital.

There are many myths about relationships, due to the various influences in society. Consider the stories shared through generations in fairytales and romantic films. Be aware that an individual might hold ideas about what a relationship 'should be' like, or what a partner 'should do', based on these influences. As Dr Russ Harris points out, there may be a belief that an individual will find that perfect partner, feel complete, find love easy, and remain in love for the rest of their life.[1] A more realistic view might be that in a healthy relationship feelings may come and go, but that individuals will act with love over time, make effort in the relationship, and continue to grow together.[2]

There are many myths about partner relationships — that there will be a perfect partner, for example, or that love should be easy. These need to be explored with couples.

There are some general principles to be aware of in relation to couple work.

- The same **communication** skills and caring apply in couple therapy as in individual therapy. The counsellor needs to be very observant when working with two individuals rather than one. Be aware of both verbal and non-verbal cues.
- **Hearing the story** of the relationship and the individuals is very important. Undertake a thorough **assessment** — this might involve seeing the couple together in the first one or two sessions, and then having one session with each individual to understand their own stories.
- It is important that the counsellor takes a very **balanced** approach in couple therapy, making it clear that each person will be treated equally and fairly.
- The counsellor will, however, need to be alert for **domestic violence**, asking appropriate screening questions. If it becomes evident that domestic violence is present — whether financial, emotional, physical or verbal — it is vital to take appropriate measures. Naming the violence and ensuring safety are priorities. Clients might need to be given information about legal aspects, community and emergency services, and be assisted in accessing them.

The counsellor needs to be alert for domestic violence, asking appropriate questions. If domestic violence is evident, it is vital to take appropriate measures.

- Create a safe space for clients to share their concerns through mindful listening, being non-judgmental and setting guidelines.
- Establish **guidelines and limits** at the outset about how the sessions will run and what is acceptable in and out of sessions; for example, how phone calls in between sessions are to be managed. For example, I sometimes suggest that anything related to appointment times, billing and so on should be discussed with the practice's administration staff, and if there is an urgent matter I will return a phone call, but that it is preferable that both partners are aware of the call. **Transparency** is important so that one partner does not feel there is collusion or bias occurring.
- Guidelines about behaviour within sessions might also need to be established, especially if there is a lot of conflict occurring. The counsellor might need to state that behaviours related to arguing, such as raised voices or rudeness, must be moderated in the session.
- As mentioned above, the counsellor might need to have an individual session or sessions with each person to hear their story and to address any individual issues. If lengthy individual therapy is needed, it is important to consider the possible options. Some couple therapists work with the individuals extensively, but my training and experience has led me to suggest individual therapists for those issues.
- Early on, it is vital to establish the **reasons** that each person has come to therapy. They might be intending to stay in the relationship and are committed to working on it, or they might have reached a stage of wanting to separate. This can be challenging as they may not have formulated this decision, or may not have communicated that they have decided to end the relationship, and so sensitivity is needed.
- Exploring the client's emotional response to what their partner is saying is vital in understanding their concerns, and to aid the partner in understanding their distress. The counsellor should acknowledge the suffering.
- Be aware that the couple might project their emotions onto the counsellor, such as anger. They might also relate to the counsellor in the same way as they relate to each other, or have related to significant others in their life, such as parents. Be aware of possible transference and counter-transference (see p. 8).

LLCC management

The early session with a couple will involve hearing the clients' stories. Questions encompass:

■ current concerns
■ current stressors
■ relationship history
■ past relationships, children and other family, including supports (genograms)
■ attachment histories with caregivers
■ individual health issues, substance use
■ social history, including interests and work
■ cultural and spiritual background
■ general health and wellbeing.

The IPT framework can assist in gathering information, via the interpersonal inventory and timeline (see p. 109). Once the history is taken, begin to formulate the BPSSC factors contributing to the current distress and identify the key issues. Although there are many differences between couples and their issues, working with couples over many years it has become apparent that many issues fall under some common headings, and these become themes which need to be addressed. The LLCC approach to couple therapy therefore focuses on the **7Cs**:

■ connection
■ communication
■ caring and compassion
■ compromise
■ conflict management
■ creativity
■ contribution and commitment.

Each of these areas will be explored later in this chapter, and the various therapies used in couple work will be integrated under each of the Cs. The 7Cs can be outlined to clients and worked through during sessions, in any order appropriate to the couple. The therapies that will be utilized most in LLCC in relation to couple therapy are **CBT**, **ACT**, **IPT** and **Narrative Therapy**, and one model not yet explored in LLCC, **the Gottman method**. More on this will follow. It might be worthwhile at this point refreshing your memory of the models outlined in Chapter 3.

Attachment theory was also introduced in Chapter 3, and it is a helpful lens for working with couples. Understanding that early attachment security in relationships with caregivers impacts on later social and emotional functioning is essential in couple work.[3] Explaining the patterns of attachment can be powerful, and that a partner might have a resultant fear of abandonment or sense of unworthiness, or a fear of being controlled, related to past attachments. This is why significant attachments, such as partner relationships, can be associated with strong emotions, especially when there is a sense of disconnection.[4]

Understanding attachment theory can enable the counsellor to interpret a client's behaviours (such as stonewalling or criticism) as reflecting this disruption. The essence of attachment theory in couple work is encouraging safe emotional connection between individuals. Fostering a secure relationship can lead to greater autonomy in a relationship.[5] In addition, attachment theory has documented some of the key interactions in couple relationships, such as the role of partners soothing each other in healthy relationships.[6]

The Gottman method

It is worth describing the Gottman method before focusing on the 7Cs. The Gottman method is based on the world-renowned work of US psychologists, Drs Julie and John Gottman. Their research focused on heterosexual marriage. However, many of the principles are useful and applicable more widely. The Gottman method teaches the couple how to become better friends and to change the ways they handle conflict. It focuses on positive interactions and developing a deep friendship involving a sense of meaning. According to Gottman, happy relationships require emotional intelligence and the key to success are **repair attempts** during and after a conflict.[7] An **emotional bank account** of goodwill is referred to, which enables the couple to give each other the benefit of the doubt. In addition, these measures lower stress levels and benefit the health and wellbeing of the individuals involved.[8]

Gottman's research has identified signs that a long-term relationship will eventually end. These include:

- Conflict being characterized by **readiness for conflict**. One partner's negativity might be so overwhelming that the other person is left feeling shell-shocked. They then disengage emotionally to protect themselves, and the fight or flight response occurs, making it impossible to have a productive conversation.
- **Failed repair attempts**, especially in combination with what Gottman names the 'four horsemen of the apocalypse', that is, **criticism, defensiveness, contempt** and **shutting down** or stonewalling.[9]
- **Rewriting the past** with a focus on the bad memories, and forgetting the happy times.
- Late signs are partners seeing the relationship problems as severe and talking things over as useless, leading **parallel lives** and loneliness.

Acceptance and Commitment Therapy

It is also worth introducing some principles from ACT in relation to couple therapy. Firstly, ACT has identified five processes that DRAIN intimacy and vitality from relationships:

- **D**isconnection — not being mindful of the other person
- **R**eactivity — not being self-aware and reacting to thoughts and feelings
- **A**voidance — retreating and distracting
- '**I**nside your mind' — getting hooked by thoughts
- **N**eglecting values.[10]

Harris has suggested the antidote to DRAIN is LOVE:

- **L**etting go of unhelpful thoughts or stories, resentment, righteousness, blaming, worrying, judging, criticizing, and being demanding
- **O**pening up to painful feelings and making changes to behaviours such as shutting down; the more the person makes room for their own feelings, the more they will be able to do this for their partner's feelings
- **V**aluing or focusing on values in relationships such as care, respect, contribution and connection
- **E**ngaging or being psychologically present, with genuine interest and openness, rather than being 'inside your mind'.[11]

The 7Cs

Having provided this background, discussion will now move back to the 7Cs and techniques from the various therapies will be introduced. Again, some will suit a particular couple more than others, and choosing the most helpful for that couple, or adapting them, is part of the art and creativity of therapy.

CONNECTION

Connection refers to **attachment** and relatedness, and encompasses being linked emotionally and physically. It is often created through small acts, such as understanding words or a gentle touch, and spending time together. When partners have been apart for the day, it is important to reconnect with eye contact, a few words, maybe briefly sharing how the day went, or a hug. This helps build trust, sets the tone for the rest of the time together, and helps prevent miscommunication and conflict.

It is important to regularly fully engage with, or give full attention to, a partner. However, over time couples tend to think they know the other person fully, may become bored and not only pay less attention to each other but also notice all their flaws. **ACT** encourages couples to be mindful of their values. The following questions can assist couples to explore their values:

- What sort of personal qualities do you want to bring into your relationship?
- What strengths do you wish to employ or develop?
- How do you want to behave or act on an ongoing basis?
- What do you want to stand for as a partner?[12]

ACT also fosters:

- a person being mindful of their partner with curiosity and openness
- asking questions that help the client see the world from their partner's point of view
- listening with the aim is of understanding, and to help the other person feel important
- letting go of unhelpful stories about the other person or the relationship.[13]

In terms of **mindfulness**, it is important to describe the concept to the couple first and explain that with couple work the aim of mindfulness is to sense what the other person is feeling. This can be done through mindful observation. Exercises to begin with include mindful hearing, breathing, seeing, tasting (such as with a sultana). Ask the couple to notice for 1 minute everything they perceive through that particular sense, and afterwards to take a moment to appreciate how that sense enriches their lives. Being mindful of one's partner can aid connection and enrich the relationship.

A further mindfulness exercise is to ask the client to become more aware of their partner's:

- facial expressions
- body language, such as hand gestures and changes in posture with different emotions
- speech — the sound of their voice, the words they use, the rhythm of their voice.

A challenging but powerful exercise is called **mindful eye-gazing**, and both clients need to be very willing to try this.

- Sit directly opposite each other, with knees interlocking.
- For the next 5 minutes, gaze mindfully into each other's eyes without talking.
- The aim is to deeply connect.
- Breathe into any uncomfortable feelings, and let thoughts float by.
- Afterwards, discuss the experience — was it hard to do, did it bring up some difficult feelings, did your mind try to distract from the task?[14]

This exercise can also be applied to hugging or cuddling, following the same steps, and expanded to **intimacy**. Intimacy involves a deep connection and the client allowing another person to really know them physically, emotionally and psychologically. Close relationships usually involve all three, but not always, and remember that each couple is unique. Intimacy needs to be consistent with values, and involves mindfulness.[15] It can be helpful to ask the couple: 'What do you value in relation to physical, emotional and psychological intimacy?' and to discuss the different types of intimacy.

- **Physical intimacy** might include having a bath together, holding hands, massage or having sex.
- **Emotional intimacy** involves a client letting a partner know their feelings. Exercises related to this might include sharing fears, having a laugh or sharing fond memories and the related emotions.
- **Psychological intimacy** refers to the client letting their partner know what is on their mind. This might related to values, goals, opinions, beliefs, desires, expectations and fantasies.[16]

Intimacy involves risk and it is important to encourage clients to take small steps, such as sharing an opinion or some of what they are feeling. Validating the other person's thoughts and feelings is vital. Clients might need to explore letting go of unhelpful thoughts and opening up to reconnecting in different ways (while at the same time practising self-care). Clients can consider connecting through words, gestures and physicality.

- **Words.** Which words might foster connection in your relationship? Examples might include 'I love you', 'I'm here for you', 'Thank you', 'I'm sorry'. Consider written words too, for example, text messages and cards.
- **Gestures.** What actions can you take, such as cooking, helping with chores, or giving gifts?
- **Physicality.** How can you facilitate connection and caring physically, for example, sitting together, hugging, kissing, holding hands, stroking, massage?

Intimacy can be fostered in many ways, and it is important to take small steps.

In addition, ACT utilizes **connection rituals**. These involve getting to know what each person finds fun and gives them joy. Perhaps there are current activities, or some done together in the past. Then several can be chosen and decisions made about doing them. Scheduling time for this, maybe a weekly movie or date night, might be helpful. Other examples are gardening or running together. It is important that each person engages fully with such rituals.[17]

LLCC TIP

Scheduling regular times to connect, through an activity or going out on a date, is important.

Understanding the other's emotional language can help a relationship, so it is helpful to talk about Chapman's **five love languages**, which proposes that individuals express their love for their partner in different ways. The languages are words of affirmation, quality time, receiving gifts, acts of service and physical touch. It is not often that a couple has the same love language, and they may become confused when their partner does not understand their communication. Awareness and practising speaking the same language can assist.[18]

An example of an exercise with the love languages is as follows:

■ Each partner identifies their own love language.
■ Then they consider which love language their partner would choose.
■ The couple then shares their answers.
■ During the next few weeks, the couple experiments with the other love languages, working up to the most important one for their partner.

In relation to connection, the Gottmans speak about making efforts to 'turn towards' a partner, that is, giving a positive response to a partner's bids for attention. These may be verbal, such as asking for attention, or nonverbal, such as a smile. Their research has shown that in strong relationships, spouses turn towards each other twenty times more than couples in distress. They say that each time a partner turns toward the other, they are making a deposit in the relationship's 'emotional bank account'. In addition, turning towards fosters more turning towards. The aim is for at least a 5:1 ratio of turning towards.[19]

Some exercises couples can do to encourage greater turning towards include the following:

■ Practise more mindfulness of how often they turn towards or away from each other.
■ Discuss positive past instances of turning towards, and opportunities for greater turning towards.
■ Choose some ways they would like the other person to turn towards them, such as a hug when connecting at the end of the day, making them

a cup of coffee or saying thank you.

- Organize time regularly to talk about something causing stress to each person. This needs to be when both individuals want to talk, and each takes about 10 to 15 minutes to talk about the stress. The other person listens, communicates interest, validates the other person's emotions, and only gives advice if asked.
- Explore times when each person has felt rebuffed or rejected. The Gottman method uses written exercises and rates the feelings. Each person can read the other's comments, and discuss the emotions and triggers. This exercise demonstrates that reality is subjective, that reactions can be based on past relationships or unmet expectations. Each person can be encouraged to take responsibility for their contribution to the situation.[20]

The Gottman method also encourages the building of a **love map**, referring to that part of the brain where the person stores all the information about their partner.[21] Gottman argues that knowledge not only fosters caring but also strength in difficult times. This is why it is important for the couple to make space in their minds for the relationship and the world of their partner. Open-ended questions are encouraged to help each person understand their partner's world. Various exercises are used, including the following, described below.

The Gottmans have devised a series of questions that partners can ask each other and see who gets the most correct, such as: 'Name my two closest friends.' 'What stresses am I facing right now?' and 'What is my favourite meal?'

LLCC TIP
Couples can have fun with some of the Gottman exercises to enhance their love map.

There is also a series of questions to encourage exploration about the other person, based on the themes of 'My triumphs and strivings; my injuries and healings; my emotional world; my mission and legacy; who I want to become'.[22]

COMMUNICATION

Most would agree that effective communication is essential in relationships. Couples regularly communicate about the time spent together and apart, money, health, gender differences (such as women potentially wanting to talk about issues and men being more process-oriented), children, family and friends. Couples often argue about these topics too.[23] Couples who present for counselling will often say communication has failed. They might mean that they are not feeling connected and able to share intimate information, and there can be communication issues such as:

- unclear communication
- not listening or being able to empathise
- dismissing partner's concerns rather than validating them
- not asking regularly about the other person's wellbeing or life
- not letting the partner know they are cared about
- presuming the partner can 'mind read' and not actually talking with them
- having expectations that the partner 'should' know about an event or issues, and not communicating about it
- not communicating about difficult topics
- not being able to express needs assertively
- not communicating respectfully
- passive-aggressive patterns of communicating
- shutting down and not communicating
- verbally abusive communication.

Note that **wanting to be in control** within the relationship can trigger some of these communication issues. This may stem from underlying unhelpful beliefs about having to be in control all of the time (to help a client further explore underlying beliefs see p. 51). It is important to discuss control in counselling, and how it can become problematic in relationships. Clients can be encouraged to reflect on how each person tries to control the other. The message to give to clients is that they cannot control each other and, in fact, the only thing they can control is their own actions.[24]

CBT can be helpful in relation to couple communication. Explaining the CBT model and unhelpful thinking patterns (see p. 130) can lead to discussion about how these may influence communication. For example, one partner might assume that they understand what the other person is thinking, or expect that the other person can read their mind. Black-and-white thinking can also influence communication, for example, one partner saying to the other: 'You always . . .' or 'You never . . .'. Jumping to conclusions can also lead to misunderstandings. However, awareness and learning to develop more helpful thinking patterns leads to less negativity and improved communication.

ACT speaks about 'asking nicely' as a means of communicating needs. It refers to unhelpful stories which may get in the way to communicating effectively, such as 'I shouldn't have to ask'. Asking calmly and respectfully is encouraged, or expressing disappointment respectfully. Practising LOVE, as outlined earlier, also opens up possibilities, such as explaining what it means to you. It is equally important to 'answer nicely': say no respectfully and yes willingly.[25]

The ways in which unhelpful thoughts then impact on behaviours related to communication can also be discussed. These might include defensiveness, eye rolling and stonewalling. Once aware, the client can then practise different behaviours. Under the banner of CBT is developing assertiveness skills, and these skills can assist clearer and more productive communication. It fosters expression of specific feelings, and identifies specific behaviours which are concerning the person. Refer to page 142 for more information on assertiveness.

IPT utilizes communication analysis with the aim of identifying incorrect assumptions, indirect verbal communication, and unhelpful silence or shutting down behaviours. The counsellor asks the client about their communication patterns, helps them to understand the effect of their communication, and works with them to establish more productive patterns. Issues related to communication sensitivities (such as shyness) or difficulties with social skills (such as in those individuals who are noted to have autism traits) may also need to be addressed via social skills training.

The **Gottman method** identifies nine skills for improving communication in couple relationships, grouped into four behaviours not to do ('the four don'ts') and five behaviours to do ('the five do's'). The four don'ts (also known as the 'four horsemen of the apocalypse') include: attacking criticism, contempt (intentional insulting and name calling, mocking, eye rolling), defensiveness (feeling injured by others in response to criticism) and stonewalling. The four do's include: calming down, complaining assertively if there is an issue (rather than remaining silent or passive), speaking non-defensively, and validating the partner by listening carefully.[26] Clients are encouraged to practise and actually *overlearn* these skills, and a useful chart can be provided to them to assist with this (see Table 21 on the next page). This table can be used to record the number of occurrences of carrying out the behaviours on each day of the week, and the total number can then be tallied. The couple can then discuss which behaviours they are achieving, or perhaps finding more difficult to manage. The chart aids understanding and also reinforces the desired behaviours.

Table 21: Gottman's nine skills for improving couple communication[27]

Behaviour	Mon	Tues	Wed	Thurs	Fri	Sat	Sun	Totals
Don't criticize								
Don't become defensive								
Don't use contempt								
Don't stonewall								
Do calm down								
Do complain (using 'I' statements)								
Do speak non-defensively								
Do validate								
Do overlearn these skills								

CARING AND COMPASSION

At the essence of caring and compassion is kindness and concern for others, and being understanding towards oneself. Relationships require these attributes, and they involve empathy and being a good friend to the other person and oneself. Relationships are then much more satisfying. **ACT**, for example, encourages appreciation of the other person and how they contribute to the relationship, beginning with mindfulness. When each person is appreciated, they are more likely to be kind to the other.[28]

The earlier mindfulness exercises can be used here (see p. 221). Following is a script for a further exercise called 'the stage show', which may also be helpful.

Imagine that you are watching a stage show. On stage is everything that you can see, hear, smell, taste, touch, feel, and think right now. Take a few minutes to notice some of the other parts of the show. For example, what your hands are doing, what you can sense against your skin, what you are thinking, what you are feeling in your body? Then bring your attention back to the room.

Mindfulness can also be applied to **appreciation** of a partner. Suggestions to enhance appreciation, and therefore caring, include asking the client to do the following:

■ Notice three things they appreciate about their partner (these can be small but important things, such as a smile or hug).

- Contemplate what their partner adds to their life, and notice ways they contribute. It is vital to appreciate the effort they make day to day.
- Reflect on their partner's strengths.
- Records can be kept about these observations and reflections, and then insights shared with their partner, such as saying 'I appreciate . . ..' or 'Thank you for . . .'.[29]

LLCC TIP

Encourage the client to practise gratitude in relationships by saying thank you, or naming three things they are grateful for in relation to the other person.

They can also be tasked with being a 'secret Ninja' — doing something nice for the other person, but secretly and with no expectation of thanks.

Caring and compassion require empathy, and acknowledging that the other person is in pain. Some people lack empathy because of their background or personality traits. Education may be needed, and practising mindfulness, helpful communication and more appreciative behaviours can assist. To get a sense of kindness for the other person, Harris suggests imagining a partner as a small child who is upset.[30] ACT suggests consciously looking at situations from the partner's perspective, and asking oneself: 'What is he/she afraid of? What does he/she want for the future? Why does this matter to him/her?' The person can then check in with their partner to see if they are correct in their thinking, for example: 'I've been trying to see things from your point of view. I'd like you to tell me if I understood correctly . . .'.

Nurturing fondness and admiration between partners is a focus in the Gottman method. The best test of this is how the couple sees the past, and the aim is for couples to detect embers of positive feelings there. This can involve appreciating the partner's positive qualities. One exercise is to identify a few positive characteristics of the partner (such as loving, intelligent, kind or practical) and sharing these, as well as recalling and sharing a time that illustrates these characteristics.[31] Discussing the history and philosophy of the marriage is also important in this regard, to remind couples of the love and great expectations that inspired their decision to marry. Use questions such as, 'Discuss how you met and got together; looking back over the years, what moments stand out?'[32]

Gottman has also devised a seven-week course in fondness and admiration based on research on the power of rehearsing positive thoughts.[33] For each day there is a positive statement or thought, followed by a task. For example, in week one each person focuses on the thought: 'I'm fond of my spouse', and also lists one characteristic they love about them. Each statement is considered and repeated throughout the day while the couple are apart.

Self-compassion is necessary if a person is to be compassionate towards others. Mindfulness, acceptance that all humans make mistakes, and treating oneself with understanding are part of this.

COMPROMISE

Remember learning about sharing as a child? You would have been taught that life is not always fair, that we need to be flexible and at times allow something to occur that is not as we would like. This was all training to be a social creature, to live with others as a member of a group. The same applies in partner relationships. Couples need to tolerate the faults of their partner and be able to compromise or make concessions and find the **middle ground**. This is often referred to as the secret of a happy relationship.

One of the myths of long-term relationships is that each person can be 'everything' to their partner. This is not humanly possible, and it is important to recognize that sometimes a need might not be able to be met by the partner, and that the individual will need to manage this themselves or in other relationships, such as friendships. CBT and Narrative Therapy can assist here, in recognizing this myth as unhelpful, and letting go of the story. Remember that the story might have come from those early fairytale influences and led to unhelpful underlying beliefs. These beliefs, along with the story, might need to be reframed.

ACT suggests drawing on the LOVE formula when there is a hard situation to resolve and compromise is necessary, namely:

- **L**etting go of resentment, blaming, judging, criticizing and being demanding
- **O**pening up to the painful feelings related to the relationship, and to the partner's feelings; acknowledging feelings is important
- **V**aluing by caring, contributing and connection; connecting with values can assist by focusing on what is important and not sweating the small things
- **E**ngaging or being psychologically present and able to focus on the partner.[34]

As mentioned earlier, clients will not always be able to have what they want. Other strategies from ACT to deal with the feelings that arise from this include:

- being mindful of the breath and focusing on the body, rather than being caught up in thoughts

- noticing thinking and naming the story, such as 'I don't deserve to get what I want'
- talking yourself through it: 'I'm so angry but I can make room for it. Breathe. Be present. I can't control how I feel, but I can control how I act.'[35]
- learning to sit with an emotion and defuse it (see the 'Being with an emotion' exercise, p. 106).

The Gottmans have carried out research into the influence of men and women in relationships, and this has an impact on willingness to compromise. Men have been found to be more likely than women to dismiss the influence of their spouse and to escalate negativity in a fight. Men who are open to influence are in the happiest, most stable relationships, and part of this has been found to be related to their wives being calmer when upset. Accepting influence encourages respect, learning, compromise, positivity and strong friendship. Men need to be encouraged to learn from their partners, as women are more oriented to discussing and understanding feelings, and are also generally more prepared for the duties involved in cohabitating.[36]

If there are challenges accepting influence, the Gottman method suggests talking about it and softening discussion about issues needing compromise, by avoiding 'the four horsemen'. Compromise involves being able to consider the other person's position, accepting influence and finding some common ground. Engaging in straightforward **problem-solving** strategies can assist (see p. 97) and other helpful strategies include 'pick a problem' and 'the paper tower'.

The couple are instructed to **pick a problem** to tackle together, then sit separately and think about the problem. On a piece of paper, each is to draw a small circle inside a larger one. In the inner circle, the person lists any aspects of the problem they feel they can't give in on; in the outer circle they list all of the aspects they can compromise on. The more open to compromise a person is, the better they'll be at persuading their spouse, so this should be reflected in the length of each list. The couple now shares their lists with each other and look for common ground. They ask:

- What do we agree about?
- What are our common feelings or the most important feelings here?
- What common goals can we have here?
- How can we understand this situation, this issue?
- How do we think these goals should be accomplished?

These steps will help the couple find a compromise. They are then to try out the solution for an agreed-upon time before revisiting it and deciding if it's working.

The 'paper tower' is a hands-on way to practise compromising together and involves building a free-standing paper tower in about 30 minutes using string, crayons, coloured markers, cellophane, newspaper, sticky tape, a stapler, construction paper and cardboard. The aim is to work as a team and to give and accept influence, and to ask questions. Have a friend rate the tower on height, strength and beauty/originality.[37]

CONFLICT MANAGEMENT

Couples who come to counselling often report escalating conflict, and assistance is required to avoid destructive escalation and to learn ways to manage conflict. Some information on conflict management has already been provided in Chapter 7, and it may be useful to refer back to this. Interestingly, the Gottmans' research indicated that most marital arguments cannot actually be 'resolved'. This is because most individuals have differences in their values, lifestyle and personality. The Gottmans talk about two kinds of couple conflict, solvable and perpetual, and that couples need to learn to identify which conflicts are solvable or which are not. The key is to identify the underlying cause of the conflict, and to practise acceptance and respect the differences. This is why the term conflict 'management' is used in LLCC rather than resolution.

Understanding the **CBT** model and being aware of unhelpful thinking patterns which may come into play as conflict escalates is important. Equally, it is important to understand that we have most control over behaviours, rather than thoughts or feelings. Encouraging helpful behaviours can assist, such as reducing criticism or stonewalling. Taking time out or walking away if need be can also be helpful behaviors. Learning to let go of the need to have the last word, and changing related behaviours, is vital.

Narrative Therapy focuses on how individuals make meaning in their lives through stories. Being aware of stories which feed conflict is a useful step in managing conflict. One example is the 'housework' story, about who is contributing more or less. Another might be the 'It is not safe to trust' story, in which the person is hyper-alert for signs of betrayal because of past experiences. These stories can be acknowledged and addressed through a narrative approach. In addition, **ACT** incorporates aspects of the narrative approach, speaking about learning to let go of some of these stories, using the following steps:

1. Name the active stories together. One might be the 'I'm right, you're wrong' story. Naming it encourages defusion of it. An exercise which encourages defusion of the story is 'a fistful of thoughts'. Ask the client to do the following:
   — Think of an unhelpful story about your partner.
   — Get all caught up in it for a while.

— Hold your hand out in front of you, and imagine taking the story out of your head and placing it on your open palm.
— Clench your fist tight.
— Slowly release the grip, open up your hand and let the story rest on your palm. Hopefully you will have experienced a sense of defusion.[38]

LLCC TIP

Harris suggests writing on one side of a card: 'I'm right, you're wrong!' And on the other side: 'Can we let go of this story and do something useful?' As soon as one person recognizes what's going on, either partner can give this card to the other.[39]

2. Sometimes couples have repeated or 'pet' arguments. An amusing metaphor can therefore be used, that of the arguments being animals! Ask the clients, 'If the recurrent arguments were animals, what sort would they be? What would they look like?' The couple can 'train' their pet arguments and also decide whether to have the pet with them or leave it behind.
3. A couple might also agree on a humorous signal or word that either person can use as a cue to let go of an argument. The couple is encouraged to be creative with this.[40]

ACT makes some other suggestions. First, after an argument, clients can consider the following questions:

■ What stories did I get caught up in? Would I like to let go of them? What feelings were problematic? Could I practise opening up to them?
■ What did I say or do to worsen things? What are some more helpful actions?
■ Did I switch onto autopilot or get stuck in my mind? How can I engage more fully and stay grounded next time?
■ Can I admit some role in the creating the conflict?[41]

ACT further suggests use of the metaphor of **taking off the armour**. If there is a difficult issue resulting in conflict, the individuals need to put down their swords and take off their armour. This means becoming vulnerable, or opening up and making space for the painful feelings. This takes courage but leads to learning and change.[42]

There has been a lot written about 'fair fighting'. ACT picks up on this concept in helpful and fun ways. It provides examples of **dirty fighting**, or tactics used to win an argument or inflict pain. Some of these tactics may be related to being in the fight or flight response and include the following:

- Springing the ambush: going off-topic and unleashing something the person did wrong in the past.
- Ganging up: getting a third party involved in the argument.
- Punching below the belt: playing on the other person's deep-seated fears.
- Playing the lawyer: twisting the other person's words, taking them out of context or exaggerating them.
- Exhuming the corpse: digging up something hurtful that happened years ago.
- Doing a silverback: throwing objects or slamming doors (beware of domestic violence in this instance).

LLCC TIP
The tactics used by the couple can be discussed and written down. It is important to maintain a sense of humour. Each person can acknowledge which ones they have used. The list can be added to by either person. Preferred tactics can then be brainstormed.[43]

Part of managing these tactics is helping the couple develop their own **ground rules**. The 'fair fighting' ground rules on page 159 can be used as prompts in discussion about the new rules. Also consider discussion based on the following: 'When we're having a fight:

- I'd like you to accept me doing this . . . I want to stop myself from doing this . . .
- I'm willing to accept you doing this . . . I want you to stop doing this . . .'

Sometimes in arguments one person will 'run' (or move away) and the other person will 'chase' them. The counsellor can help the couple understand these behaviours, exploring the feelings involved with questions such as:

- Why do you run? How do you feel when you run? On the other hand, how do you feel if chased?
- How do you feel if your partner runs? Why do you chase? How does chasing feel?

Attachment patterns can be explored and empathy encouraged by asking each person to say what they think it must be like for the other person. Alternative behaviours can then be discussed.

Individuals and couples dealing with difficult emotions, such as anger or hurt during conflict, need to be able to soothe themselves, and each other. To **self-soothe**, allow at least 20 minutes to calm yourself down. Let your partner know that you are feeling overwhelmed and need some time out. Then practise some mindfulness or meditation. **Soothing each other** follows, once individuals are feeling calm. Talk about it, and then have a cup of tea together or give the other person a shoulder massage, for example.

Resentment can build up over years in relationships. Harris calls this 'psychological smog', or the thoughts, feelings and memories which erode the relationship. ACT invites the couple to consider various layers of smog and what effect they have on the relationship. The layers include:

- the 'should' layer, for example, 'She should apologize'
- the 'no point trying' layer — 'It's too late, there's too much damage'
- the 'if only' layer — 'If only he would get his act together'
- the painful past layer — dwelling on bad memories
- the scary future layer — 'He'll just do it again'
- the reason-giving layer — 'I'm too stressed'
- the judgment layer — 'He doesn't deserve to be treated well'
- the 'I know why' layer — 'She's doing it on purpose to hurt me'
- the deep-seated fears layer — 'I'm not good enough for her'.[44]

It is important to recognize such thoughts; they may or may not be true, and may not be helpful. An individual cannot prevent all such thoughts but they can control their response. Thoughts do not create the smog, but holding on to them does. Exercises include discussing smog in couples, and identifying old and new thoughts which contribute.

ACT also picks up on Gottman's repair attempts (more on this later in this chapter), and the importance of **forgiveness**. Resentment can build up in relationships for many reasons and eat away at positive feelings. If one person is left (or perceives they are left) to do the housework or child-rearing, or one person believes they sacrificed their career for the other person, resentment can arise. Forgiveness can relieve related suffering, but is challenging at times. It is important to remember that forgiveness does not involve forgetting or excusing, but it does involve LOVE (see p. 229).[45]

Forgiveness does not mean **trust**. If there has been a breach of trust in a relationship, such as through gambling or **infidelity**, trust must be rebuilt and this takes time. With significant breaches of trust, the partner who has broken the trust must be willing to explore their actions, personality, beliefs and lifestyle, to see what has contributed. The couple needs to look at the relationship and any problem areas. Sometimes individual as well as couple work is helpful.[46]

Trust must be earnt again via the other person's actions, including speaking honestly and being reliable. Amends may need to be made. In developing trust, it is best to focus on trusting in small ways first, and seeing if the trust is deserved. Gradually, larger actions of trust can be taken. As trust is re-established, self-protective actions will become less necessary. Acceptance is required — that you can never be certain that the partner will not repeat the behaviours — but that they are committed and making effort.

When the **IPT** assessment identifies 'interpersonal disputes' as a problem area, the counsellor works with the couple to learn ways to manage them. The disputes might include overtly hostile conflict (such as domestic violence, verbal abuse), betrayals (infidelity, conflicting loyalties), disappointment or general conflicts. The goals in IPT are to identify dispute/s and to make choices about a plan of action. This may include modifying communication patterns, reassessing expectations or looking for ways to satisfy needs outside the relationship. As mentioned earlier, it is important to know whether each person is committed to working through the disputes or not.

Useful questions to consider are:

- What are the chief issues in the dispute/s?
- What are differences in expectations/values between the client and the other party in the dispute?
- What are the client's/other party's wishes in the relationship?
- How has the client resolved disagreements in the past? Can those techniques be used here, or are new ones needed?
- What are the strengths/weaknesses of the relationship?
- What are the client's options?
- What resources does the client have to bring about change in the relationship?
- What changes are realistically possible?

Management strategies which can be used in IPT include:

- finding parallels in previous relationships
- exploring what the client gains from their behaviour
- having an optimistic tone about the potential for change
- brainstorming strategies and ideas with couple
- utilizing techniques such as communication analysis, improving communication skills, teaching expression of emotion and role-play.

Conflict management may end with resolution of the dispute or acceptance of relationship limitations. Conflict may ultimately lead to the end of relationship.

A powerful technique from IPT is working with particular incidents of conflict. The incident is explored to collect information regarding any miscommunication, and to raise insight and encourage change. Let's take the story of Chris and Leanne. They came to a session having had an argument over the previous weekend. If this had not been the case, the counsellor could have begun the conflict discussion by asking: 'Tell me about the last time you had an incident . . .'. Using the grid in Table 22, the counsellor takes the couple through the incident in stages:

1. First, the counsellor picks up on general statements about the incident.
2. Then they enquire about the effect or emotion generally.
3. More specific details are then sought about the incident.
4. Finally, the effect is explored in more detail.

Table 22: The IPT conflict grid

Exploring interpersonal disputes	General statement	Specific incident
Content	1. Describe incident: 'She isn't interested in me . . .	3. Gather more information: 'It was Saturday night, we had a nice dinner, but she couldn't wait to get home and do some work . . .'
Effect	2. Describe the effect: 'I felt hurt.'	4. Clarify effect further: 'I felt hurt and very angry.'

Once this information is obtained, the counsellor and the couple then consider whether expectations were clearly communicated or not, and what styles of communication were used. They can brainstorm other possibilities for managing the situation, and redo the grid using other general statements. A pro forma for the table to use in working through incidents if provided in the Appendix (see p. 302).

The **Gottman** method highlights the importance of making **repair attempts** in relationships. These attempts can involve words or actions aimed at repairing the relationship after conflict. Practice is often needed to use them and recognize attempts at repair. Focusing on the words being used can help, for example, sentences beginning with 'I feel' or 'I appreciate' may be a repair attempt, or statements such as 'I need to calm down', 'Can we take a rest' or 'Sorry'. Asking for a truce, acknowledging pointlessness, using empathy or apologizing can be repair attempts. At the start, couples can be encouraged to let the other person know that they are making an attempt or accepting an attempt.[47] Sometimes humour can help, too.

LLCC TIP
Brainstorming ways to make 'repair attempts' can be helpful.

Earlier in this chapter, the Gottmans' work on solvable versus perpetual conflict was highlighted. Couples can get into gridlock over some issues, for example, whether to have children or which location to settle in. Although some issues might not be solvable it is important to talk about them as they can involve dreams, and an individual might not think their dream is being respected. Frustration and hurt can occur, and emotional disengagement can result. Research has shown that couples who feel happier appreciate that understanding the other person's dreams or viewpoints is vital, as is helping each other realize dreams. Compromise and acceptance may be needed.[48]

CREATIVITY

Creativity can help relationships to not only survive but to flourish! It can help in dealing with problems through creative problem-solving and lateral thinking. It can be used to instil some fun and flexibility into relationships, and to revive intimacy. Creativity can be applied to appreciating each other and finding new ways to express this, and applying 'the five love languages' can be enhanced through creativity.

A good starting point is **Gottman**'s work on creating shared meaning in relationships. This might involve:

- revisiting values
- exploring the culture of the couple's relationship or family, looking how things are done and if there are particular customs or rituals; an example would be how birthdays are celebrated
- asking whether and how partners support each other's dreams
- exploring any spiritual dimensions to the relationship
- sharing the stories of each individual in the relationship.

Note that couple or family **rituals** are a great way to connect and build identity as a unit. These might be as simple as eating dinner together, having movie nights, opening presents together on birthdays and having a special celebration, getting together with friends or the couple having regular date nights. Romance can be woven into this to foster intimacy. In sessions, the couple can plan rituals and begin to make them regular events.

CONTRIBUTION AND COMMITMENT

Healthy relationships require both contribution and commitment by partners. Both require effort. As mentioned earlier in this chapter, some of the common topics discussed by couples — and a common cause of stress and conflict — are time spent together and apart, money, health, and gender differences which influence the relationship. Addressing these issues through the lens of contribution and commitment can help the relationship.

A starting point is to consider how the couple views their different roles in the relationship, because this will influence contributions made. This discussion can also clarify expectations of each person. **CBT** can be helpful in relation to understanding unhelpful thinking about expectations of the partner. Underlying beliefs may need to be explored and addressed, such as 'being taken for granted'. It can also be helpful to talk through the couple's goals, individually and together. Values can drive these goals, and working together on shared goals can increase contribution.

Connecting with each other and learning to soothe each other when one is stressed can be an important contribution to the relationship. This requires commitment, and soothing might involve kind words or actions. With specific areas such as finances, the couple should talk about concerns and work on budgeting together. Be mindful of long-term goals to work towards as a couple. Home duties, such as housework and cooking, often need to be reviewed to ensure each partner is contributing fairly; making decisions about who will do which tasks can help. Equally vital is working through who will contribute what to the care of a new baby or children.

The need to determine whether partners are committed to staying in the relationship has already been highlighted. Using a scale of 0 to 10 for degree of commitment can clarify the level of commitment. It can be helpful to discuss that commitment involves effort and making changes. It also involves acceptance of what cannot be controlled or changed. The more couples focus on what is in their control, the more empowered they will feel. Interestingly, when the focus shifts to what can be controlled, partners often start to spontaneously make positive changes.

ACT encourages clients to clarify and act on values to be the partner they want to be, to manage the painful feelings, and to stop acting in ways that impact negatively on the relationship. Once the decision has been made to commit to the relationship and work on it, LOVE is needed. LOVE can also be applied to working on sexual intimacy. As a reminder, LOVE involves:

■ **L**etting go of unhelpful thoughts, stories, resentment, blaming, criticizing etc.

■ **O**pening up to painful feelings and making changes to behaviours

■ **V**aluing or focusing on values such as caring and contribution

■ **E**ngaging or being psychologically present, with genuine interest.[49]

The Gottman method speaks about maintaining relationship momentum in five 'magic' hours per week. This practice, outlined below, requires contribution and commitment.

1. With partings, ensure that before saying goodbye in the morning you've learnt about one thing happening in your spouse's life that day (2 minutes a day x 5 working days = 10 minutes per week).

2. On reunion, discuss stressful events from the day (20 minutes a day x 5 working days = 1 hour 40 minutes).

3. Show daily admiration and appreciation for your partner (5 minutes a day x 7 days = 35 minutes).

4. Show affection each day, for example, kiss your partner before sleep (5 minutes a day x 7 days = 35 minutes).

5. Have a weekly date and update love maps and turn towards each other (2 hours once a week).

Commitment may involve being involved in couple counselling for a period of time or intermittently. It may also involve **Bibliotherapy** and reflecting. The books by Harris, the Gottmans and Chapman are very helpful. These therapists/authors also have websites with useful information. See 'Resources' for more information.

In summary

Relationships can bring great joy, and also great stress! How individuals behave in relationship can reflect their earlier attachments. When individuals or couples present for counselling for relationship issues, the LLCC approach focuses on the 7Cs: connection; communication; caring and compassion; compromise; conflict management; creativity; contribution and commitment.

Effort is required to work on relationships, and there are many helpful tools and strategies to utilize. It may take LOVE or letting go of unhelpful thoughts, feelings and behaviours; opening up to painful feelings; focusing on values such as caring and respect; and engaging or being interested and present. It is important to make attempts to repair the relationship after conflict, and to practise forgiveness.

Reflection on Chris and Leanne's story

Chris and Leanne both reported being committed to working on their relationship. More information was gathered in the early sessions, and the counsellor had an individual session with each of them. Leanne described how in her family, there was a lot of noise and talking. If there was an issue it was sorted out, often with yelling. Chris shared how he lived in fear of his father as a child, and how he feared that if became very angry, he might be like his father.

Sessions focused on the 7Cs, with an emphasis on conflict management. Chris and Leanne became more empathic about each other's behaviours and they both worked on modifying their behaviours in conflict situations. They found helpful the discussion about soothing each other when distressed, expressing more appreciation of each other, and connecting through some enjoyable activities.

Leanne expressed her concern about Chris's business, and he made efforts to let her know how it was going and to reassure her that he would close it down if finances deteriorated. They talked about short- and long-term financial goals. The relationship became more solid as time went on and they acted on their commitment. In the end they decided to move in together.

LLCC TIPS: HEALTHY RELATIONSHIPS

- Connect regularly.
- Appreciate each other and the small things.
- Communicate feelings.
- Keep intimacy alive.
- Know the other person well.
- Manage conflict constructively.
- Have shared goals and respect each other's dreams.
- Problem-solve regularly.
- Be creative in relationships.
- Put in effort and contribute.
- Make a commitment to the relationship.

Resources

Books

Cassidy, J. and Shaver, P. 2008, *Handbook of Attachment: Theory, research, and clincial applciations*, The Guilford Press, New York.

Chapman, G. 2010, *The 5 Love Languages: The secret to love that lasts*, Northfield Publishing, Chicago.

Gottman, J. M. and Silver, N. 2007, *The Seven Principles for Making Marriage Work*, Orion, London.

Harris, R. 2009b, *ACT with Love*, New Harbinger Publications, California.

Websites

National Coalition Against Domestic Violence, United States: www.ncadv.org

Information on IPT: www.interpersonalpsychotherapy.org

New Zealand Women's Refuge: www.womensrefuge.org.nz/WR/Domestic-violence/Domestic-violence.htm

Pro formas from Harris (2009), *Act with Love*: http://www.actmindfully.com.au/free_resources

ReachOut.com, Australia: au.reachout.com/tough-times/bullying-abuse-and-violence

Relationships Australia: www.relationships.org.au

South African Police Service, domestic violence information: www.saps.gov.za/resource_centre/women_children/domestic_violence.php

The Gottman Institute: www.gottman.com

White Ribbon Australia's campaign to prevent men's violence against women: www.whiteribbon.org.au/

Women's Aid, United Kingdom: www.womensaid.org.uk

Phone apps

Breathe2Relax: http://t2health.dcoe.mil/apps/breathe2relax

Breathing Zone: www.breathing-zone.com

Meditation Oasis: http://www.meditationoasis.com/apps/

Smiling Mind: www.smilingmind.com.au

Chapter 13
Building self-belief

What lies behind us and what lies before us are tiny matters compared to what lies within us.

—RALPH WALDO EMERSON

Many clients struggle with their sense of self-worth. They may say, 'I have low self-esteem' or they might be highly self-critical. Firstly, consider as a person or as a counsellor whether you have experienced your own thoughts about not being 'good enough' and whether these thoughts undermine your confidence. Whether thinking about clients or yourself, this chapter is all about ways to deal with self-doubts and enhance self-belief. Read Ronan's story and as you read the chapter, reflect on what strategies might assist him.

Ronan's story

Ronan is a 23-year-old university student. He is struggling with feelings of anxiety and low mood. During early meetings with his counsellor he talks about doubting his abilities, and says he has always had low self-esteem. Ronan finds that he constantly compares himself to his friends and other students, and has high expectations of himself. He is very self-critical and expresses some of these thoughts in counselling sessions, such as, 'I never seem to be as good as the other students in tutorials'.

Background

With clients like Ronan, it is important to explain some of the terms related to self-belief that we commonly use. In LLCC the preferred terms are self-belief and self-compassion. Here are some of the main ones.

- **Self-esteem** refers to how the person sees and judges themselves, often in comparison to others. It describes self-opinion and sense of **self-worth**.
- Self-esteem affects how the person functions generally and how they relate to other people. It includes **self-confidence** or how confident a person feels about their abilities.[1]
- The person's underlying beliefs about themselves, when constructive, are referred to as **self-belief**, and these drive thinking about oneself and self-confidence.
- A more recent term is **self-compassion**, which means that the person is kind and understanding towards themself when faced by personal failings, instead of criticizing and judging themselves harshly.[2]
- The term **self-acceptance** (accepting our mistakes and letting go of self-judgments) is also used.[3]

Low self-belief can affect health and wellbeing in many ways, so addressing it can assist the client. Low self-belief can contribute to stress, anxiety and low mood. In turn these can affect sleep and eating habits, or the ability to exercise. It can be tiring and distracting for the client focusing on their limitations, and low self-belief can affect their coping behaviours, such as engaging in leisure activities. Low self-belief can affect the client's self-confidence and may prevent them from socializing or going to work functions. It may affect assertiveness with others, or cause the client to avoid putting themselves forward for tasks at work through fear of failing.

Low self-belief can contribute to stress, anxiety and low mood. In turn these can affect sleep and eating habits, or the ability to exercise.

The LLCC approach highlights the influence of life experiences and society on the client. Let's consider these influences and self-belief.

- **Early life experiences:** A child who experiences a lot of criticism growing up, for example, will struggle to develop a strong sense of self-belief. The child might take on the belief that they are not 'good enough' or that they don't achieve what is expected of them.

- **Ongoing life experiences:** Experiences in families, relationships or in the workplace continue to influence self-belief. The negative and intimidating behaviours of a bully or abusive individual, for example, will impact on self-belief. Compare these people to encouraging individuals who boost self-belief.

- **The society in which we live:** The potentially positive or negative influences of media, culture, government and education, for example, have been outlined earlier. Women, for example, might take on the view that to be worthy they must be attractive, nurturing, smart, successful and more. Men might take on the idea that they also must have certain attributes, such as being strong and successful. These views tend to be unrealistic and can lead to the client putting pressure on themselves through comparison with an unrealistic ideal.

LLCC also recognizes the influence of human biology and personality. Humans tend to compare themselves to others as a survival mechanism. In the modern age, comparisons may not be so much about survival but comparison still occurs, including to people showcased by the media or 'friends' on Facebook. Comparing to others with terms such as winner, loser, failure, champion creates 'a fragile basis for self-esteem'.[4] It is helpful to point out to clients that often what they see of others is just a snapshot of their lives, with areas of life screened out from view. In addition, we live in a world in which success is often defined by material possessions or notoriety, and this can be lead to another comparison trap.

Cognitive Behaviour Therapy

For a client to feel or act more confidently, they might need to do some work on their thinking or underlying beliefs. Some of the underlying beliefs that can rob the client of self-belief include:

- 'I must keep proving myself through my achievements.'
- 'I must be 100 per cent competent.'
- 'I must do things perfectly.'
- 'I must have everyone's approval.'
- 'I need to be loved to be worthwhile.'
- 'The world must be fair.'[5]

Perfectionism can drive the client to have high expectations of themselves and a sense of not doing well enough if not meeting those expectations. It is hard to have a strong sense of self-belief if those expectations are getting in the way. Equally, a sense of wanting to please and looking for approval from others can challenge self-belief. Consider, too, whether the client is an optimistic thinker. Optimistic thinking can help the client focus on positive events in their life and their strengths, whereas negative thinking can contribute to low self-confidence. Negative or perfectionistic thinking can be black and white i.e. 'That went really, really well' or 'That went really, really badly', rather than seeing possibilities in between.

It is helpful to talk through the following points with clients:

- Our worth is not actually about what is achieved. Achievements give a sense of satisfaction, but not true self-belief, and involve focusing on the future rather than the present.
- Perfectionism is sometimes useful in helping achieve our goals and to do well, but it is not always helpful and can lead to procrastination, anxiety and disappointment.
- Humans seek approval from others, but it is important not to base the measurement of self-worth on the expectations or the praise of others. What is really important is what the client thinks about themselves, whether they accept themselves and what they do.
- Humans feel a deep need to be loved, and in fact most people are loved by others. It is important not to base self-worth on being in a partner relationship.
- Unfortunately there is suffering in the world and things are not always fair. Clients won't always get what they would like, and so talking about being realistic and flexible is useful.

Self-worth is not actually about what is achieved, nor about what others think.

Here are some strategies from CBT to utilize with clients around self-belief. Discuss them with clients, and help them work through the strategies step by step.

- Identify unhelpful self-critical thoughts, such as, 'I can never do anything right'. Keeping a thought diary can assist (see p. 99).
- Educate the client about unhelpful thinking traps, and then assist them to identify any unhelpful thinking or thinking traps, for example, over-generalizing or being too black and white. Encourage them to watch out for critical self-labels (such as 'I am hopeless').
- Help the client challenge their thinking by asking them, 'What is the evidence for the thought?' or asking themselves, 'Am I being too harsh?' Encourage them to look for exceptions to their thoughts ('I did manage to achieve . . .') and to avoid critical labels.
- Finally, ask them to consider more helpful thoughts, such as, 'Actually, I do a lot of things very well' and 'I work hard and do my best'.[6]

A technique that has proven useful over many years in clinical practice comes from *Recovery of Your Self-Esteem: A guide for women* by Carolynn Hillman and is equally applicable to both men and women. It involves three steps for the client to follow:

1. **Recognize your positive points** by making a list of: 'What I like about myself: my positive points'. This list can include any attributes or behaviours viewed as positive, such as being a good cook, being punctual or being a kind friend. The client might wish to ask others for ideas and it is recommended they read the list regularly.
2. **Recognize the 'inner critic'** or the inner negative voice and make a list of: 'Things I do not like about myself: negative points'. In addition, consider whose voice is being critical — has the criticism been internalized from other people in the client's life?
3. Then **reassess** these negative things and be fairer on yourself — in other words, work on self-belief. Are the statements too critical? Can they be reworded so they are less harsh? Try reframing the statements into goals — an example would be reframing the statement 'I have no confidence in front of others' as 'I tend to be quiet in front of others, but I am working on my confidence and on talking with people more'.[7]

Acceptance and Commitment Therapy

ACT encourages the client to identify the main causes of low self-belief or self-confidence, such as high expectations of self, self-criticism, pre-occupation with fear or lack of experience. It offers a framework for the issues which keep self-belief low, using the acronym FEAR:

- **F**usion
- **E**xcessive goals
- **A**voidance of discomfort
- **R**emoteness from values.

ACT then DAREs the client to move forward with self-belief through:

- **D**efusion
- **A**cceptance of discomfort
- **R**ealistic goals
- **E**mbracing values.[8]

This framework can be explored with the client, and if they want to make changes to their self-belief a good starting point is writing a **life change list**.[9] The client can complete this list, keep it in their diary or wallet to refer to often, and start with small actions. Table 23 outlines a life change list.

Table 23: Life change list

As I develop self-belief . . .

Here are some ways I will act differently:

. . . .

. . . .

Here are some ways I will treat others differently:

. . . .

. . . .

Here are some ways I will treat myself differently:

. . . .

. . . .

Here are some personal qualities and character strengths I will develop and demonstrate to others:

. . . .

. . . .

Here are some ways I will behave differently in close relationships with friends and family:

. . . .

. . . .

Here are some ways I will behave differently in relationships involving work, education, sport or leisure:

. . . .

. . . .

Here are some important things I will 'stand for':

. . . .

. . . .

Here are some things I will start or do more of:

. . . .

. . . .

Here are some goals I will work towards:

. . . .

. . . .

Here are some actions I will take to improve my life:

. . . .

. . . .

Russ Harris writes about the role of fear in holding us back from self-belief. He says that having self-confidence is not about absence of fear, as fear can be a source of energy, but about changing our relationship with fear.[10] We can experience fear or anxiety as emotions, memories, images, thoughts or sensations. It is important to guide the client to lessen the struggle and fusion with these, and to help them be aware of thoughts that the mind generates about not being able to do something, for example, predictions something won't go well or harsh self-judgments.[11] The client can then challenge themselves to do the task, despite the mind presenting barriers.

In relation to these thoughts, what matters is not whether the thoughts are true, but whether they're helpful. It is easier to let thoughts come and go than to eliminate them. ACT encourages the client to ask themselves: 'If I allow this thought to guide my actions, will it help me create the life I want?' They can manage the thoughts with ACT defusion or letting-go techniques, which involve noticing when stuck in unhelpful thoughts, naming this as being '**hooked again**' and neutralizing the thoughts by techniques covered earlier. For example, saying to themselves 'I'm having the thought that . . .' or 'Thanks brain for that thought' using a silly voice or singing the thought out loud (see p. 106).

LLCC TIP
Questions from ACT can be helpful to manage self-depreciating thoughts. An example is the question: 'If I allow this thought to guide my actions, will it help me create the life I want?'

To assist the use of these techniques in day-to-day life, encourage the client to experience several **defusion** exercises. These techniques take practice and the client works with the one/s they find most useful. Once these skills are developed, it is easier to defuse from thoughts spontaneously.

An example of an ACT defusion exercise to enhance self-belief follows:

- Pick a self-judgmental thought, fuse with it and notice how you feel. Then replay the thought but this time first say to yourself, 'I'm having the thought that . . .' followed by 'I notice I'm having the thought that . . .'. Notice your reactions.
- Replay the thought and say, 'Thanks, mind, for sharing that thought.'
- Pick another self-judgmental thought, fuse with it and notice how you feel. Now say the thought with a silly voice, or sing it to the tune of 'Happy Birthday' or another tune. Notice your reactions.
- Use the metaphor of 'leaves on a stream' — imagine placing each thought on a leaf and allow them to flow gently down a stream.[12]

Another ACT technique follows, which has similarities to the reframing exercise by Hillman but focuses more on defusion from critical thinking. The counsellor guides the client to acknowledge their negative thinking, such as 'I'm fat' or 'I'm stupid', by writing these thoughts on one side of an index card. This is named the 'bad self'. Positive thoughts such as 'I'm kind and a good friend' are named the 'good self' and written on the other side of the card. The client is asked to read each side and to get caught up (or fused) with those thoughts. They are then asked to put the card on their lap and notice that as long as they let it sit there it doesn't matter what side of the card faces up, it does not stop them from doing what they want to do. The counsellor also gives the client homework to take the card and write down more points on each side during the week, and to read both sides each day. The result is less fusion with self-judgments.[13]

One of the key aspects of the ACT model is committed **action**. Applied to self-belief, it is important to remember that actions of confidence are the first step and feelings of self-confidence will follow. This can be thought about as 'acting confidently'. Practising new skills is also vital. It is also important to base actions on values, as this helps shift the emphasis away from the outcome to engaging in the process and gaining from it.[14] Values can be discussed with the client and they can identify the ones most important to them. This leads into discussion about the life domains as outlined in Chapter 2. The client can work through these domains and consider what is important in relation to each domain and where there are some gaps. Focus particularly on those that might be related to a low sense of self-belief. Then set some short-term and longer-term goals driven by values rather than achievement.

To overcome the fear which can arise in relation to these goals, suggests there is a need to tolerate some unpleasant feelings. Take the client through the 'Being with an emotion' exercise (see p. 106) so they have a strategy to use to manage any fear that arises. Another approach when fear shows up is to:

- allow it — notice and acknowledge it, plus make room for it
- befriend it — welcome it, be pleasant and affectionate towards it, collaborate with it
- channel it — make use of the energy it gives you.[15]

Sometimes clients will have failures as they work towards their goals. This is part of life, and we can learn from this experience. Remind the client that as long as they have acted on their values, then even if the goal is not achieved they have still been successful and received feedback to enable them to take further action.[16] Harris provides some useful tips for managing failure:

- Unhook from unhelpful thoughts.
- Make room for painful feelings.
- Be kind to yourself, in word and gesture.
- Appreciate what worked and appreciate any improvements.
- Find something useful to help you learn and grow.
- Take a stand through acting on your values.[17]

In summary, ACT teaches the client that:

- the actions of confidence come first; the feelings of confidence come later
- genuine confidence is not the absence of fear; it is a transformed relationship with fear
- 'negative' thoughts are normal, and it is important to defuse them rather than struggle with them

- self-acceptance is key
- true success is living a life consistent with values
- don't obsess about the outcome; become passionate about the process
- failure hurts — but if you're willing to learn, it's a wonderful teacher.

Mindfulness

Mindfulness in its own right can assist the person struggling with self-belief to relax and be more involved in the moment. We spend a lot of our lives living mindlessly, so paying attention to the moment helps us connect to ourselves, others and the world. It helps us focus on the now instead of the past or future, and to be less judgmental. In particular, it helps the client to be mindful of their thoughts and feelings, noticing them rather than getting caught up with them. Through mindfulness the client can learn that thoughts and feelings come and go, and that they can experience greater calm and peacefulness. In this way mindfulness can assist in developing self-acceptance and **self-compassion**.[18]

> Through mindfulness the client can learn that thoughts and feelings come and go, and greater peacefulness can be experienced. In this way it can assist in developing self-compassion.

Consider a person who is socially anxious and needs to attend a work function or social engagement. They may feel very nervous and get caught up with their thoughts such as: 'Everyone will think I am boring and that I have nothing to say' or 'What if I say the wrong thing and they laugh at me?' Mindfulness can be utilized to focus on the moment, on the breath, or on listening to what others are saying rather than ruminating.

Interpersonal Therapy

Social skills training from IPT can also be helpful in learning to make conversation and be more assertive. A colleague once said that when she feels low and lacking in self-esteem, she focuses on what it is like to be feeling better and more confident. This gets her back to feeling more positive. Sometimes she pretends she is feeling confident and this helps lift her, too.

Narrative Therapy

The central stories in our lives was discussed earlier, and of particular relevance in this chapter is that we attempt to understand ourselves by creating stories in our mind. If we have some negative stories dominating our lives (such as 'I'm not worthy'), Narrative Therapy can help us to view ourselves differently. Remember that clients will have many strengths and will have survived many challenges. Sometimes a client will focus on a dominant story, such as 'I am not good enough', rather than the exceptions to this, that is, the times they have done well and achieved things, even in very small ways or the fact they have been a survivor and overcome challenges.

LLCC TIP

Ask the client to consider one story about themselves they would like to reframe and give it a name. Then take the client through narrative questioning (see p. 111) about that story. Help them rewrite the story.

Positive Therapy

Seligman, the founder of Positive Psychology, states that Positive Psychology (PP) is the psychology of PERMA — **p**ositive emotion, **e**ngagement, positive **r**elationships, **m**eaning and positive **a**ccomplishment.[19] Building our capacity in all of these key areas enables us to not only feel good but to develop our resources and discover new skills and ways of being, including building our self-belief. Positive self-esteem is viewed as a predictor of wellbeing.[20] Our thinking plays a key role in this.

To assist clients to build self-belief, PT encourages a focus on strengths and using them more. It has been shown that if the client gets to know and use their strengths and abilities, they will develop greater confidence.[21] Discuss strengths with clients using Table 24 on the next page. See if they relate to any of the strengths listed and discuss.

Table 24: Strengths[22]

Action	Innovation
Adventure	Judgment
Authenticity	Legacy
Catalyst	Listener
Change agent	Mission
Compassion	Moral compass
Competitive	Optimism
Courage	Order
Creativity	Persistence
Drive	Personal responsibility
Emotional awareness	Persuasion
Empathic connection	Planner
Enabler	Rapport builder
Explainer	Relationship deepener
Gratitude	Resilience
Growth	Scribe
Humility	Self-awareness
Humour	Service
Improver	Time optimizer
Incubator	Work ethic

Following are some other ideas for working with strengths:

- Encourage the client to look at www.authentichappines.sas.upenn.edu and complete the strengths survey to discover more information about their strengths.
- Ask the client to write down three of their signature strengths, and then look at three ways they use them. Can they think of new ways to use them?
- Ask the client to write a list of three activities that use some of their strengths. They can then choose one to participate in during the next week.
- Get hold of some strengths cards and have them in your office — you can lay them out on the desk or floor and the client can choose ones that apply to them. Ask them to find examples from their lives of times when they displayed or used these strengths.

In addition, the following strengths knowledge scale can be used. It indicates levels of knowledge of personal strengths and the likelihood of using them.

Table 25: Strengths knowledge scale[23]

Rate each statement below from 1 to 6 (1 = disagree; 2 = slightly disagree; 3 = neither agree nor disagree; 4 = slightly agree; 5 = agree; 6 = strongly agree)

1. Other people see the strengths I have.
2. I have to think hard about what my strengths are.
3. I know what I do best.
4. I am aware of my strengths.
5. I know the things I am good at doing.
6. I know my strengths well.
7. I know the things I do best.
8. I know when I am at my best.

Scoring: Start by subtracting your score for question 2 from 8 (e.g. if you scored 5 for question 2, then 8 – 5 = 3). Now add this figure to the responses fo each of the items. A higher score indicates a higher level of strengths knowledge. People who use their strengths are more likely to be able to use them and be effective in doing so.

Engagement in **activities** and **social relationships** has many benefits, such as positive emotions, positive relationships and having a sense of accomplishment. These can also contribute to building self-belief. Engaging in activity can help us find meaning and a sense of purpose, and I saw much evidence of this when working as an occupational therapist early in my career. One woman who had had a stroke and was depressed was encouraged to engage in an activity that was of value to her, which was helping her son. She fixed up the old number plate from her son's car for his 21st birthday, and in the process her sense of purpose in life and mood improved.

Gratitude is one of the positive emotions that PT highlights and encourages. It means different things to different people; it might, for example mean thanking someone or 'counting your blessings'. In addition, it can evoke a feeling of wonder and an appreciation of life. It is good to practise gratitude as it has been found to be an antidote to negative emotions such as worry and irritation, and people who experience gratitude have been shown to be happier, more energetic and more hopeful. Gratitude allows us to embrace positive life experiences, taking from them maximum satisfaction, and expressing gratitude reinforces self-worth and self-esteem — appreciating how much others do for us and how much we achieve ourselves gives us greater confidence. Gratefulness takes the focus away from the negative aspects of the client's life and places it on what is valued. A simple way to foster gratitude is to encourage the client to keep a gratitude journal. Note that the optimum time to write in a gratitude journal is once a week.[24]

LLCC TIP

Encourage clients to keep a regular gratitude journal. Once a week the client writes down three things they are grateful for, no matter how small. Gratitude phone apps can also be used as a way of highlighting what you are grateful for.

Eleanor Roosevelt wisely said, 'No one can make you feel inferior but yourself'. This is why it is helpful to foster a sense of **self-compassion**. This means the client is kind and understanding towards themselves when faced by personal failings, instead of criticizing and judging harshly.[25] There are a number of elements to self-compassion, including the following:

- Having compassion means that we offer kindness to others when they make mistakes. Likewise, self-compassion involves acting the same way towards ourselves when we are having a difficult time.
- Self-compassion means we choose to care for ourselves instead of judging, being self-critical and comparing ourselves to others.
- It means that we are kind and understanding when confronted with personal mistakes. We all make mistakes as we are human!

In other words, encourage the client to apply the Golden Rule to themselves — to treat themselves as they do others, with kindness and understanding! It is also important to put things into perspective rather than buying in to comparisons. The things that are really important are health, connecting with others and having meaningful activities to engage in. It can be helpful to ask the client to record times when they are kind to themselves, and bring this record in to a counselling session.

The following script for a **loving-kindness meditation** can be useful for clients.

Make yourself comfortable and let your eyes close. Focus your attention on the breath and relax a little more with each breath out.

> *Relax your body from the top of your head, down to the tips of your toes. Then focus on the region of your heart. Get in touch with your heart, and reflect on someone for whom you feel warm, tender and compassionate feelings. This could be a child or partner, or a pet. Visualize or imagine yourself being with this loved one and notice how you feel. Extend loving-kindness to them by saying: 'May you be well, may you be at ease, may you be happy and at peace.' Hold on to the warm and compassionate feelings.*

> *And now extend those warm feelings to yourself. Extend kindness to yourself as you do others, and allow your heart to radiate with love. When you are ready, open your eyes and bring your attention back to the room.*[26]

Hypnotherapy

Hypnotherapy can assist in building self-belief through the wide use of ego-strengthening, which has long been used as a way of helping clients to enhance their self-confidence and self-worth. It involves giving repeated suggestions about self-confidence or self-worth, with the theory that they are then held in the person's subconscious mind and exert an influence on their thoughts and feelings. Examples of direct ego-strengthening suggestions are: 'You will feel more calm and confident each day' or 'You will become more aware of your strengths as time goes on and tap into them each day.' Indirect suggestions can be also be used, such as: 'As you sit and look out over the valley, you gain a different perspective about life and, in particular, about yourself and your abilities.'

Milton Erickson, a famous American psychiatrist (1901–1980), used many indirect suggestions and metaphor. He developed a technique of looking at a positive experience in the client's past related to feelings of pride and self-worth, and linked these feelings to the client's current life. The technique of **anchoring** is similar to this and is now widely used. The therapist asks the client to think about a time when they felt very confident, to get in touch with that experience and the feelings, and then to lock those feelings into the mind by squeezing together the thumb and index finger of their dominant hand. Whenever the client then wants to get in touch with those feelings, all they need do is squeeze together those fingers.[27]

There are many hypnotherapy scripts available related to ego-strengthening; some examples follow.

INSTILLING POSITIVE EXERCISE

Make yourself comfortable and let your eyes close. Focus on the breath and relax. Using all of your senses, imagine being in the countryside or at the beach. Find a spot to sit or stand near the water, and notice there are some pebbles or shells on the ground around you. Gather some of them up and feel them in your hand; see their colours and feel their textures.

Your mind is like the water: the conscious part of the mind is like the water's surface, while underneath the surface is like the unconscious. Now take your time and attach positive meaning to each of the pebbles or shells. One might represent confidence or trust in your intuitive abilities; another might represent looking after yourself. Then, one by one, toss them into the water. Know that they will penetrate the surface of the water and float down until they settle on the bottom. In the same way, these ideas will settle into your mind. When you are ready, gradually open your eyes and return to the here and now.[28]

TREE MEDITATION

Imagine you are standing next to a beautiful tree with strong roots, a broad trunk and leafy branches spreading upward. Notice the colours of the tree, the textures and the smell. The tree is not only beautiful, it is amazing. It has weathered many storms and continued to grow strong and tall. It takes what it needs from the environment — water, sunshine, nutrients, carbon dioxide — and it gives back oxygen and shelter . . .

When you consider it, you are a lot like the tree. You have many strengths, you take and you give back. But you are more than the tree as you can move, think and feel.[29]

Hypnotherapy can be a vehicle for visualizing positive events and success. We can see this in sport. Watch Olympic finalists before a race or a dive; they can be seen focusing, in trance, visualizing successfully completing their event. It is also used by musical or stage performers to build confidence and self-belief. Suggest clients use visualization before social or work events; they can take a few moments to picture the event going well from beginning to end.

We can develop our self-awareness through noticing our internal state, mood and thoughts, by reading books, watching films or documentaries, talking with others, journalling, meditation, reflection or prayer, travelling, personal development courses, further study, creative activities, being in touch with nature (for example, gardening or walking in a park or at the beach) or undertaking psychotherapy. Many clients find using affirmations is powerful for them. These are positive statements in the present tense, such as 'I am feeling more confident each day' or 'I am being kinder to myself in my mind'. Affirmations can be written on cards and left in places that the client will see each day, such as on the fridge or bathroom mirror. Reading them regularly helps create new ways of thinking.

LLCC TIP
Direct the client to imagine a circle, a bit like a hula hoop, on the ground in front of them. This is their circle of self-belief. Then ask them to get in touch with a time when they felt a strong sense of self-worth or self-confidence, and then to step into the circle. Suggest to them that stepping into the circle will intensify the feeling tenfold. They can repeat this a few times, and repeat whenever they want to. They might want to jump into the hoop as they start to feel more confident![30]

Intuition

The concept of **intuition** can be discussed with clients in relation to self-belief, as it can help individuals to feel more confident about themselves and their decision-making. Humans often move between rational and intuitive thinking when making decisions, and in work settings. Intuitive information is received through the senses and bodily feelings, or intuitive thoughts or hunches might occur. Intuitive skills can be enhanced through awareness and practice. Seven steps to develop intuition were outlined on page 13 and further information can be found in Howell (2013), *Intuition: Unlock the power!* Central is trusting heart-felt knowledge, as the client is the expert on themselves and they have strengths, knowledge and intuition.[31]

Bibliotherapy and e-mental health

There are a number of useful books listed in 'Resources' at the end of this chapter, and look out for chapters on self-belief in the various CBT texts. Several websites are also highlighted.

In summary

If I could have a dollar for all the clients I have seen for whom self-belief is an issue, I would be very wealthy! Clients frequently express that they do not perceive themselves as 'enough'. This chapter has provided understanding as to why this is such an issue for people, and also provided many ways for counsellors and clients to work on this. It will be well worth the effort, as the enhanced self-belief will influence so many other aspects of the client's life. And if they can treat themselves more compassionately in the future it will prevent many difficulties from arising.

Let's consider Ronan's story again, and hear about what assisted him to develop his self-belief and to feel more confident at university.

Reflection on Ronan's story

Ronan and the counsellor focused on his high expectations of himself and how they were working for and against him. The trap of comparison to others was discussed, and the CBT model explained. Ronan did a thought diary and was surprised how self-critical his thinking was. The concept of self-belief was discussed, and Ronan was very interested to learn some mindfulness techniques. He read widely around this topic, and really took on the concept of self-compassion. In fact, he decided to do an assignment about it.

LLCC TIPS: BUILDING SELF-BELIEF

- Work might be needed on changing thinking and underlying beliefs about oneself, and quitting overly self-critical thoughts.
- Change unhelpful stories, such as 'I am not good-enough'.
- Focus on values, accept what is not within your control, and take action that helps create a meaningful life.
- Practise mindfulness as opposed to being caught up in thoughts or feelings. This leads to more calmness and self-compassion.
- Focus on strengths, positive emotions and purpose/accomplishment.
- Enhance relationships and connect with others.
- Accept compliments — just say thank you!
- Stand tall and smile, and celebrate success.
- Remember to trust heartfelt knowledge or intuition.

Resources

Books

Harris, R. 2009, *ACT Made Simple: An easy-to-read primer on Acceptance and Commitment Therapy*, New Harbinger Publications, California.

Hillman C. 1992, *Recovery of Your Self-Esteem: A guide for women*, Simon & Schuster, New York.

Howell, C. 2009, *Keeping the Blues Away: The ten-step guide to reducing the relapse of depression*. Radcliffe Publishing, Milton Keynes.

Howell, C. 2013, *Intuition: Unlock the power!* Exisle Publishing, New South Wales.

Howell, C. and Murphy, M. 2011, *Release Your Worries: A guide to letting go of stress and anxiety*, Exisle Publishing, New South Wales.

Seligman, M. 2011, *Flourish: A visionary new understanding of happiness and wellbeing*, Random House Australia, Sydney.

Tanner, S. and Ball, J. 2001, *Beating the Blues: A self-help approach to overcoming depression*, Doubleday, Sydney.

Websites

ACT Mindfully: www.actmindfully.com.au

Dr Cate Howell, blog, resources on self-belief: www.drcatehowell.com.au

University of Pennsylvania, Authentic Happiness, strengths questionnaire: www.authentichappiness.sas.upenn.edu/search/node/strengths%20 questionnaire

3 FURTHER LLCC KEY FOUNDATIONS

The little reed, bending to the force of the wind, soon stood upright again when the storm had passed over.

—AESOP

Part 3 focuses on two key or foundational areas in counselling: firstly, crisis intervention, and secondly, 'more than self-care' for the counsellor. This title for Chapter 15 has been coined as counsellors are well aware of the need for self-care, but the aim will be to explore some new ideas and other layers to self-care.

A range of people might be involved in crisis intervention, including hospital and emergency staff, mental health professionals and counsellors. I have been involved in crisis intervention over the years in different capacities — as a doctor in hospital and community settings, working with the military, and as a therapist. According to researcher, J. Mitchell (2015), the goals of crisis intervention are to reduce the impact of an event and to assist recovery.

The crisis that counsellors are most likely to encounter in practice is seeing the client who is suicidal. Therefore the focus of Chapter 14 will be on suicide prevention. Chapter 15 will then focus on practising self-care as a counsellor, which is vital given the issues they will potentially be hearing about and dealing with.

Chapter 14
Crisis intervention

Crisis management refers to methods used to offer immediate help to individuals who have experienced an event that produces significant distress. It focuses on short-term strategies to prevent damage, and can be followed by longer-term counselling.[1] The principles include:

- being calm, empathic and supportive
- keeping your response simple, immediate and practical
- setting up expectations of a positive outcome.[2]

The way the counsellor communicates with the client is key in managing the crisis. A calm manner, support and reassurance are vital. The focus of this chapter will be on the 'here and now' issues, the client's safety, and establishing a plan for managing the crisis. In managing a crisis such as suicidality, the counsellor needs to be aware of their duty of care, which involves ensuring a client does not come to foreseeable harm by their actions or failure to act.[3] Counsellors must also be mindful of any risk posed to other individuals by the client. It is essential for counsellors to document their actions and choices.

Simon's story

Simon is 24 years of age. He has seen a counsellor called Alex in the past to help with stress and symptoms of anxiety. He calls Alex's office in crisis on a Friday afternoon, as his girlfriend of two years broke off the relationship earlier in the week. He is feeling very distressed and anxious, and is not sleeping. He is tearful and says to Alex that he does not see the point in being alive now, and just wants to not feel so bad. He is scared that he will harm himself, and has thought about taking paracetamol. He has not harmed himself in the past and has a supportive family.

Background

Background information on suicide is provided in this chapter, as this informs management of the suicidal client. First, some facts about suicide deaths.[4]

- Every year a significant number of suicide deaths occur worldwide, with approximately 2500 each year in Australia, 40,000 in the United States and 5700 in the United Kingdom.[5,6]
- The highest age-specific suicide rates occur for males in the 85+ and 80+ age groups, followed by the 45–49 age group; and for females, the 80–84 age group, followed by 50–54 and 15–19 age groups.
- More males than females die by suicide, and in Australia the rates for Aboriginal and Torres Strait Islander people are twice those of non-Indigenous Australians.

There are a number of factors associated with suicide:

- mental health conditions (such as Major Depression, Bipolar Disorder and Schizophrenia)
- substance use disorders
- acute stresses such as relationship breakdown, grief or financial crisis
- prolonged stress factors, such as bullying, unemployment or domestic violence
- long-term issues related to childhood abuse
- serious chronic health issues or pain
- previous suicide attempts
- family history of suicide.[7]

It is important to be aware of the following:

■ Asking a client about suicidal behaviour will not cause the client to commit suicide. They will often be relieved that the question has been asked as there can be fear, shame or guilt associated with suicidal thinking.[8]

■ In general, increases in frequency, intensity and duration of suicidal behaviour are an indicator of severity.[9]

■ **Red flags** in relation to risk include the client talking about killing themselves, having no reason to live, being a burden to others or being in unbearable pain. Behaviours may also change, such as increased risk-taking behaviours, substance use, withdrawing from people and activities or giving away possessions.[10]

■ With suicide, people talk about 'feeling suicidal' but it is more accurately described as a thought about how to solve perceived inescapable problems.[11] The feelings are often overwhelm, hopelessness and psychological pain, with a sense of isolation from others, and suicide is seen as a way to not continue to feel these feelings.[12]

Asking a client about suicidal behaviour will not cause the person to commit suicide.

Guidelines

General guidelines include the following points:

■ Talk openly and non-judgmentally.

■ Be collaborative and offer assistance.

■ Know your legal and ethical responsibilities.

■ Be aware of risk factors for clients.

■ Conduct an assessment, including risk assessment.

■ Obtain previous risk assessment information if possible.

■ Honestly determine your own competencies — if necessary seek more training or hand over care to an appropriate professional.

■ Consult with colleagues.

■ Consult with family members, carers, significant others if appropriate.[13]

■ Determine areas that assistance may be offered during and after the crisis.

■ Post-crisis, the client may be assisted by a range of therapies, such as CBT,

ACT and IPT, depending on their situation and issues; learning to tolerate emotional distress can be an important part of the counselling process.

Assessment

There is a useful resource called SQUARE. It says that asking appropriate questions in the right way, at the right time could save a life.[14] It encourages the counsellors to:

- **engage** effectively — offer assistance, provide the opportunity to talk; be aware that there might be past mental health problems such as depression
- **respond** — be open to and respectful of the client's experiences and feelings, and listen with full attention; use open questions initially and don't be afraid to ask specific questions
- **be aware** — create a stigma-free environment; it is unhelpful to argue or criticize.[15]

A systematic approach to the client who is suicidal is vital. Be aware of background issues, including past suicide attempts and mental health problems. However, the focus is on the current crisis. Listen to and explore thinking about suicide. A simple scaling question — 'How effective would suicide be as a way to solve your problems?' — asked after problems leading to suicidality have been described will give you this important information (on a scale of 0 to 5, with 1 meaning not effective and 5 meaning extremely effective). Those who have strong beliefs that suicide will solve their problems are at greater risk.[16]

A basic, but helpful, suicidality assessment tool follows in Table 26.

Table 26: Suicidality assessment tool[17]

To assist in assessing suicidal risk, ask the following questions of the client with respect to the last month:

1. 'Do you want to harm yourself?'

2. 'Have you thought about suicide?'

3. 'Have your made any plans to take your own life?' If yes, ask for specific details.

4. 'Have you attempted suicide?' This refers to more recent attempts.

5. 'At any time in life have you ever attempted suicide?'

It is generally regarded that questions 2, 3, 4 and 5 are more strongly indicative of suicidal risk. Suicidal risk accelerates with an increasing number of 'yes' responses. However, if the client responds with 'yes' to any of the questions then it is vital to carefully assess the suicidal risk and organize psychiatric involvement if necessary.

SQUARE ASSESSMENT

Based on the SQUARE resource and suggestions by Consultant Psychiatrist Dr Randall Long, there is a series of questions which may be asked as part of the assessment.[18] Importantly, the questions should be asked **in the sequence in which they are presented below**; and note that each affirmative response indicates that the next question should be asked.

1. Suicidal thoughts

- Passive — 'Do you wish you didn't have to go on living? Do you have thoughts of wanting to die?'
- Active — 'Do you have thoughts of wanting to take your own life? Do you have suicidal thoughts?'

2. Suicidal threats

'Do you to talk with others about killing yourself? Have you told anyone that you were going to kill yourself?'

3. Suicide plans

'Have you ever thought about methods to kill yourself?'

4. Suicidal plans: the details

- Decision — 'Have you decided on a method to kill yourself?'
- Details — 'Have you made a plan of exactly what you might do to kill yourself?'
- Resistance — 'Have you been able to resist carrying this out? What stopped you putting the plan into action?'
- Preparations — 'Have you started preparations to suicide?'
- Time profile — 'For how long have you had the plan? Have you set a date to kill yourself?'
- Affairs — 'Have you put your affairs in order? Have you made arrangements for after you die? Have you written a note?'

OTHER RISK ASSESSMENT TOOLS

Two more detailed standardized risk assessment tools include the Modified Scale for Suicidal Ideation and the Columbia Suicide Severity Rating Scale.

The clinician-administered **Modified Scale for Suicidal Ideation**

(MSSI) developed by Miller et al. is a tool in the public domain that can assist in risk assessment. It consists of eighteen questions which assess the presence and severity of suicidal ideation. If a low score is received on the first four questions there is no need to administer the full scale. The scale considers the client's thoughts and actions over the last 48 hours. A total score is calculated, resulting in a rating of low, mild or severe suicidal ideation.[19]

The **Columbia Suicide Severity Rating Scale** (C-SSRS) is used widely across the world and has been found to lead to a significant reduction in suicide attempts. It has subscales which address presence and severity of ideation, intensity of ideation, behaviours (such as harm to self, dangerous actions, preparatory acts) and lethality. This scale requires training — more information can be found at www.cssrs.columbia.edu/training_cssrs.html

CLINICAL INTUITION

In addition to the more formal assessment, be aware of **clinical intuition**. It can play a valuable role. For example, if the client is saying that they are 'fine now' and your intuition is indicating that they are not, listen to it. Experience has reinforced how important clinical intuition can be.

LLCC management

The key principles of management are ensuring safety in the first instance (this might involve referral to emergency mental health services or removing means — for example, tablets or any weapons), addressing underlying issues and providing continuity of care. It can be helpful to draw up a collaborative management plan including:

- client details
- identified stressors/issues to be addressed
- management goals and steps
- who is responsible for which steps (and in what timeframes)
- relapse, including warning signs.
- follow-up.

Ongoing review is vital as relapse can occur. Remember that contracts drawn up between client and counsellor are *not* helpful, and can lead to a false belief the client will be safe. A useful summary of the assessment and management of suicide risk is presented in Figure 13.

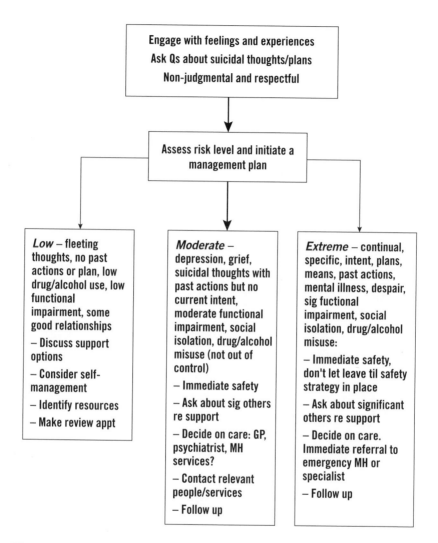

Figure 13: Assessment and management of suicide risk[20]

In summary

This has been a brief overview about the crisis intervention and, in particular, the assessment and management of the client who is suicidal. This is a challenging area and training, experience and supervision will assist. Resources are provided for further information. Now let's reflect on Simon's story.

Reflection on Simon's story

Alex makes time to see Simon. He is very distressed, and Alex has a supportive and open discussion with him. He gathers some background information but focuses on the crisis. Alex runs through a series of questions about suicidal thinking and planning, and more information comes to light. Simon's thinking is focused on suicide and he has a strong desire not to be in emotional pain.

Simon has made plans to buy paracetamol to take on the weekend, and has formulated a suicide note in his mind. Alex expresses concern and empathy, and explains that he has a duty of care to ensure Simon's safety. Simon is willing to receive help, as he is frightened by the intensity of his thoughts. He agrees to wait while Alex phones the local mental health triage number, and Alex is instructed to organize an ambulance for Simon to attend the nearest emergency department.

Rather than tips on managing suicidality, following are tips for counsellors working in areas in which they may manage clients who are suicidal.

LLCC TIPS: FOR COUNSELLORS MANAGING SUICIDALITY[21]

- Undertake education on managing clients who are suicidal, and on the impact of this work on counsellors.
- Learn from peers through case discussion (both formal and informal).
- Utilize appropriate supervision.
- Practise management by working through a case (this may relieve anxiety when faced with instances in the field).
- Plan ahead, and find out what is expected from counsellors in different organizations and settings, and what procedures are in place for support.
- Be mindful of personal safety needs.
- Understand professional and personal limits, and monitor work or case load.

Resources

Books

Chiles, J. and Strosahl, K. 2004, *Clinical Manual for Assessment and Treatment of Suicidal Patients*, American Psychiatric Publishing, Virginia.

Websites

American Foundation for Suicide Prevention: www.afsp.org

Beyondblue: www.beyondblue.org.au

Centers for Disease Control and Prevention, suicide link: http://www.cdc.gov/violenceprevention/suicide/definitions.html

Columbia Suicide Severity Rating Scale: www.cssrs.columbia.edu/training_cssrs.html

Living Is For Everyone (LIFE): www.livingisforeveryone.com.au/

New Zealand mental health resource: http://www.mentalhealth.org.nz/get-help/a-z

NHS, suicide information: http://www.nhs.uk/conditions/suicide/pages/introduction.aspx

NHS, self-harm information: http://www.nhs.uk/conditions/self-injury/pages/introduction.aspx

South African Depression and Anxiety Group: www.sadag.org

Suicide Questions Answers Resources (SQUARE): www.square.org.au

Chapter 15
More than self-care

Take rest; a field that has rested gives a bountiful crop.

—OVID

Counselling can be amazing work, and it can be draining. Counsellors will have contemplated self-care many times during their training, but being in the field brings the need for self-care — or more than self-care — into perspective. This chapter will highlight some of the important aspects of self-care and hopefully provide new ideas to contemplate and perhaps put into action.

Remind yourself about Alex's story. He was able to assist Simon in a compassionate and competent way; but consider now how his work has had an impact on him.

Alex's story

Alex graduated as a counsellor 12 months ago. He is gradually building up his practice and sees a lot of young people. Simon, a client in his twenties, presents on a Friday afternoon, saying that he has broken up with his girlfriend of two years and cannot see the point in living. The client is very distressed, and Alex offers support and begins to assess and deal with the situation.

It has been a difficult few weeks for Alex, in practice and in his own life. Alex has seen a number of clients with challenging issues, and one in particular impacted on Alex. The client had shared their story of being sexually assaulted at a beach 6 months previously.

In his own life, Alex was dealing with some relationship issues and wondering whether the relationship would continue.

Background

Counselling work can take its toll on individuals, at times generating stress and exhaustion. Working with trauma in particular can involve many emotional challenges and trigger compassion fatigue characterized by symptoms of chronic stress.[1] **Vicarious traumatization (VT)** — trauma reactions in counsellors resulting from exposure to clients' traumatic experiences — can also occur.[2] This will impact on the counsellor's wellbeing, their work and relationships, and is associated with higher rates of anxiety and depression, substance use and suicide. Given counsellors often have strengths of empathy, caring, kindness or compassion, they are perhaps more vulnerable to these issues and care is needed to maintain the counsellor's wellbeing.

Symptoms and signs of VT include:

- emotional numbing
- social withdrawal
- nightmares
- feelings of despair
- more negative view of the world
- loss of sense of spirituality
- loss of enjoyment in activities
- reduced respect for clients
- tiredness
- sense of cynicism

- increased absenteeism
- reduced motivation
- difficulties in relationships.[3]

LLCC management

It is reported that:
- three ways to protect yourself from VT are awareness, balance and connection
- three ways to address VT are self-care, self-nurturing and escape
- three ways to transform VT are challenging negative beliefs, finding meaning and participating in community building.[4]

Some of these ideas will be incorporated as more general self-care measures are explored. This chapter aims to increase awareness about self-care and counsellors may decide to undergo further professional development in this area. Learning from peers and supervisors is also very valuable. It is important that the counsellor consider themself in a holistic way, being aware of their physical, emotional, social and familial, intellectual, occupational, cultural, aesthetic and spiritual needs. To help others, the counsellor needs to function at relatively high levels in each of these areas.

A good place to start is to undertake the **self-care assessment** in the Appendix (see p. 303). This will give you an idea of how well you are caring for yourself in the different aspects of your life. A balanced and meaningful personal life is essential to helping others, and this comes back to you living a life consistent with your values.

LLCC TIP
Undertake the life domains values exercise in Chapter 2 for yourself (see p. 33). Consider what is important to you in each of the domains and if there are any gaps or imbalances currently. This will help you identify any areas in your life which need some attention.

Another way to look at what is important to you is to imagine that you have only 12 months to live. What would you do with that time, and would it be good to do more of it now?

Counsellors are encouraged to engage in their own personal self-care activities. It is important to practise what you preach and model self-care and a healthy lifestyle to clients, and looking after your wellbeing is vital. Here are some ideas:

- Eat well and sleep well.
- Exercise regularly, including both incidental and planned exercise, as any movement is good!
- Drop multitasking some of the time.
- Practise mindfulness as much as possible each day (including in sessions with clients).
- Use meditation regularly or learn self-hypnosis.
- Keep a personal journal or gratitude journal.
- Tap into optimistic thinking and positive emotions.
- Appreciate others and the world.
- Enhance self-belief.
- Think creatively and enjoy creative activities.
- Connect with others and allow time for friends and family.
- Take mini-breaks and holidays regularly.
- Find meaning in life and purpose; maybe tap into spirituality.
- Learn from the various therapies such as CBT and ACT. Apply the principles in your own life.
- Practise kindness and **self-compassion** (more on this later).

In relation to work practices, it is important to follow the guidelines below.

- Monitor self-care
- Monitor for signs of VT.
- Use mindfulness at the start of a session with a client — to benefit the client and counsellor.
- Be organized, and manage time effectively.
- Take a few minutes between clients.
- Leave life pressures at the office door when starting the day, and leave the pressures of work in the room on leaving. Rituals can help with this, such as making a list of things to follow up the next day before leaving the office.
- Diversify work and case load.
- Learn to communicate assertively.
- Delegate tasks, such as administrative or accounting tasks.
- Be a reflective counsellor, and if a session with a client is challenging reflect on reasons for this. Do not ignore emotional reactions; sit with them and use mindfulness or ACT techniques to manage the reactions. Talk with a peer or supervisor if necessary.
- Check yourself for any resentment, judgment or generalizations towards

clients and discuss with your supervisor. These reactions are quite normal but need to be examined honestly in order for you to grow and to maintain a non-judgmental attitude. Burnout can result if not managed.

■ Recognize and acknowledge your strengths, where you did well, where you feel you may have made a difference in a client's life or feel uplifted after a session.[5]

SELF-COMPASSION AND MINDFULNESS

One of the key messages of the LLCC approach is practising self-compassion — being kind and understanding towards oneself when faced by personal failings, instead of criticizing and judging oneself harshly. Self-compassion has been shown to be associated with happiness, optimism, wisdom, curiosity and emotional intelligence. It can also help us deal with pain and help our relationships.[6]

As outlined previously, there are a number of elements to self-compassion:

■ Having compassion means that we offer kindness to others when they make mistakes. Self-compassion involves acting the same way towards ourselves when we are having a difficult time.

■ Self-compassion means we choose to care for ourselves instead of judging and being self-critical, and comparing ourselves to others.

■ It means that we are kind and understanding when confronted with personal mistakes. We all make mistakes as we are all human!

Self-compassion involves accepting our negative emotions as part of life and being willing to observe our negative thoughts and emotions in mindful awareness. Mindfulness is a non-judgmental and open-minded state in which one observes thoughts and feelings as they are, without trying to suppress or deny them. Mindfulness also requires that we don't fuse or overidentify with our thoughts and feelings, so that we are caught up and swept away by them.[7]

Now apply this concept to yourself and your practice. As a counsellor, remember to treat yourself as you do others: with kindness and understanding. It is also important to put things into perspective rather than comparing yourself to other counsellors. Also aim to practise more mindfulness in your day-to-day life and in practice. It can enhance your wellbeing and your work.

You might like to use the following **loving-kindness meditation** for yourself:

Make yourself comfortable and let your eyes close. Focus your attention on the breath and relax a little more with each breath out. Relax your body from the top of your head down to the tips of your toes. Then focus on the region of your heart. Get in touch with your heart, and reflect on a loved one for whom you feel warm, tender and compassionate feelings. This could be a child, partner or a pet. Visualize or imagine yourself being with this loved one and notice how you feel. Extend loving-kindness to them by saying: 'May you be well, may you be at ease, may you be happy and at peace.' Hold onto the warm and compassionate feelings. And now extend the warm feeling to yourself. Extend kindness to yourself as you do others, and allow your heart to radiate with love.

When you are ready, bring your awareness back to the room, and open your eyes.[8]

In summary

Counselling can be very rewarding but can also generate stress and exhaustion. Vicarious traumatization can also occur. This will impact on the counsellor's health, work and relationships. Self-care measures are important to maintain the counsellor's wellbeing. Counsellors are encouraged to engage in their own personal self-care activities, such as eating healthily, meditating and enjoying leisure activities. It is also important to practise what you preach and model self-care to clients. Counsellors are also invited to embrace mindfulness and self-compassion or, in other words, to extend the same kindness to themselves as they do to others. This is all part of caring!

Reflection on Alex's story

Alex managed the situation with Simon competently. However, that weekend he kept thinking about the client and reflecting on whether he had taken the correct actions, and about his other clients. He found it hard to relax and decided to talk with his supervisor the following week.

Alex and his supervisor talked about the clients, and reflected on the degree of trauma Alex was hearing about from his clients. The supervisor also asked what was occurring in Alex's own life. Alex talked about the stress he was under in his own relationship, and also made a connection between Simon and himself in terms of relationship issues.

The supervisor asked about self-care. Alex had been working hard recently and had not had as much time to exercise or catch up with friends. He decided to allocate more time to this and to plan a weekend away. He also reminded himself to practise more mindfulness at work and home.

To complete this chapter, and the book, and to encourage you in your caring role, it is fitting to provide some tips on self-compassion, and to extend the Buddhist loving-kindness poem to you as a counsellor:

May you be filled with loving-kindness
May you be well
May you be peaceful and at ease
May you be happy

LLCC TIPS: SELF-COMPASSION

- Apply the golden rule to yourself and treat yourself as you do others: with kindness and understanding!
- Quit self-criticism: let go of being too self-critical.
- Use kind words — avoid labels such as 'hopeless' or 'useless', or anything else that is negative.
- Use affirmations involving positive and compassionate sentiment.
- Practise mindfulness or being in the present moment, which allows us to be more accepting.
- Remember that you are human, and drop comparisons with others.
- Smile on the outside as well as the inside!
- Look after your body — eat well, sleep well and exercise.
- See that our perceived weaknesses can also be our strengths.
- Put things into perspective and be grateful.

Resources

Books

Fredrickson, B. 2009, *Positivity: Ground-breaking research to release your inner optimist and thrive*, One world Publications, London.

Germer, C.K. 2009, *The Mindful Path to Self-compassion: Freeing yourself from destructive thoughts and emotions*, Guilford Press, New York.

Gilbert, P. 2009, *The Compassionate Mind*, Constable, London.

Hanh, T.N. 1997, *Teachings on Love*, Parallax Press, Berkeley.

Harris, R. 2009, *ACT Made Simple A quick-start guide to ACT basics and beyond*, New Harbinger publications, California.

Lyubomirsky, S. 2007, *The How of Happiness*, Sphere, London.

Websites

ACT Mindfully: www.actmindfully.com.au

Dr Kristen Neff, self-compassion information: http://www.self-compassion.org/what-is-self-compassion/definition-of-self-compassion.html

Positive Psychology Center: www.ppc.sas.upenn.edu
Your Guide to Mindfulness-based Cognitive Therapy: http://www.mbct.com/

Phone apps

Breathe2Relax: http://t2health.dcoe.mil/apps/breathe2relax
Breathing Zone: www.breathing-zone.com
Meditation Oasis: http://www.meditationoasis.com/apps/
Smiling Mind: www.smilingmind.com.au

Appendix

1. K10 test[1]

Indications	<ul><li>Screening scale for mental disorders</li><li>Measures non-specific distress</li><li>Good guide to a mental disorder</li></ul>
Limitations	For general indications of 'mental health'. Clinicians still need to make own judgment if patient needs treatment.
Scoring tips	<ul><li>Likert scale (1, 2, 3, 4, 5) for each question</li><li>Maximum score 50</li></ul>
Cut-off scores	<20 normal 21–24 mild 25–29 moderate 30+ severe
Comments	<ul><li>2 minutes to score. 25% of people presenting in primary care will have a score of 20 or over. If post-treatment scores are over 24, consider referral to specialist.</li><li>Based on the last 4 weeks.</li><li>Patient to fill out.</li></ul>

Name: .... Date: ....

Please indicate how you have felt by placing a number between 1 and 5 in the space provided to the right of each statement

1	2	3	4	5
none of the time	a little of the time	some of the time	most of the time	all of the time

1. In the past 4 weeks, about how often did you feel tired out for no good reason? ☐

2. In the past 4 weeks, about how often did you feel nervous? ☐

3. In the past 4 weeks, about how often did you feel so nervous that nothing could calm you down? ☐

4. In the past 4 weeks, about how often did you feel hopeless? ☐

5. In the past 4 weeks, about how often did you feel restless of fidgety? ☐

6. In the past 4 weeks, about how often did you feel so restless you could not sit still? ☐

7. In the past 4 weeks, about how often did you feel depressed? ☐

8. In the past 4 weeks, about how often did you feel that everything was an effort? ☐

9. In the past 4 weeks, about how often did you feel so sad that nothing could cheer you up? ☐

10. In the past 4 weeks, about how often did you feel worthless? ☐

K10 = ☐

2. Depression Anxiety Stress Scale (DASS)

	DASS
Indications	Assess quantitative scores for depression, anxiety and stress in out-patient population.
Limitations	Assess, not to replace diagnostic judgment.
Scoring Tips	Use transparency sheet. Add 7 'A', 'D' & 'S' items separatley, then double the score obtained. Refer to z scores if you wish.

Cut-off Scores		Depression	Anxiety	Stress
	Mild	10–12	7–9	15–17
	Moderate	13–19	10–14	18–25
	Severe	20–26	15–19	26–33
	Extreme	27+	20+	34+

Comments	Scores depression, anxiety and stress in one test. Reliably correlated with Beck scale. Australian norms used, good scale. 3 scores in one test. *Patient to fill out.*
Reference	Lovibond, S. & Loviboind, P. (1995). *Manual for the Depression Anxiety Stress Scales.* Psychology Foundation of Australia Inc. Sydney, NSW.

Name: .... Date: ....

Please read each statement and circle a number 0, 1, 2 or 3 which indicates how much the statement applied to you **over the past week**.

The rating scale is as follows:

       0 Did not apply to me at all

       1 Applied to me to some degree, or some time

       2 Applied to me to a considerable degree, or a good part of time

       3 Applied to me very much, or most of the time

1.	I found it hard to wind down.	0	1	2	3
2.	I was aware of dryness in my mouth.	0	1	2	3
3.	I couldn't seem to experience any positive feeling at all.	0	1	2	3
4.	I experienced breathing difficulty (e.g., excessively rapid breathing, breathlessness in the absence of physical exertion).	0	1	2	3
5.	I found it difficult to work up the initiative to do things.	0	1	2	3
6.	I tended to overreact to situations.	0	1	2	3
7.	I experienced trembling (e.g., in the hands).	0	1	2	3
8.	I felt that I was using a lot of nervous energy.	0	1	2	3
9.	I was worried about situations in which I might panic and make a fool of myself.	0	1	2	3
10.	I felt that I had nothing to look forward to.	0	1	2	3
11.	I found myself getting agitated.	0	1	2	3
12.	I found it difficult to relax.	0	1	2	3
13.	I felt downhearted and blue.	0	1	2	3
14.	I was intolerant of anything that kept me from getting on with what I was doing.	0	1	2	3
15.	I felt I was close to panic.	0	1	2	3
16.	I was unable to become enthusiastic abot anything.	0	1	2	3
17.	I felt I wasn't worth much as a person.	0	1	2	3
18.	I felt that I was rather touchy.	0	1	2	3
19.	I was aware of the action of my heart in the absence of physical exertion.	0	1	2	3
20.	I felt scared without any good reason.	0	1	2	3
21.	I felt that life was meaningless.	0	1	2	3

S = [   ]   **A =** [   ]   **D =** [   ]

DASS Scoring Template

S

A

D

A

D

S

A

S

A

D

S

S

D

S

A

D

D

S

Multiply each sum by 2

D =

A =

S =

A

A

D

DASS Profile Sheet

Name: . . . .   Date: . . . .

Age: . . . .   Sex: . . . .

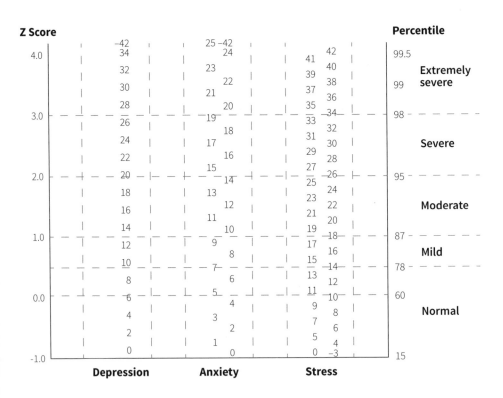

For each scale, draw a horizontal line through the score obtained for that scale, and fill in the dotted lines below to form a bar graph. The heights of the bars are in Z score units and may be compared with each other and with the severity labels. Note that conversion to percentiles on the right-hand axis is approximate only.

3. HEADSS adolescent health check[2]

Client name	
Date of visit	
Date of birth	
Other services/adults involved in client care	

PSYCHOSOCIAL ASSESSMENT, HEADSS FRAMEWORK

H — Home
(Consider: living arrangements, transience, relationships with carers/significant others, community support, supervision, abuse, childhood experiences, cultural identity, recent life events)

E — Education, Employment, Eating, Exercise
(Consider: school/work retention and relationships, bullying, study/career progress and goals, nutrition, vegetarianism, eating patterns, weight gain/loss, exercise, fitness, energy)

A — Activities, Hobbies and Peer Relationships
(Consider: hobbies, belonging to peer group, peer activities and venues, lifestyle factors, risk-taking, injury avoidance, sun protection)

D — Drug Use
(Consider: alcohol, cigarettes, caffeine, prescription/Illicit drugs and type, quantity,
frequency, administration, interactions, access, recent increases/decreases, past
treatments, education, motivational interviewing)

S — Sexual Activity and Sexuality
(Consider: sexual activity, age onset, safe sex practices, same sex attraction, history
pap smears/STI screening, sexual abuse, pregnancy/children)

S — Suicide, Depression and Mental Health, Safety/Risk
(Consider: normal vs clinical depression, anxiety, reactions to stress, risk assessment
if appropriate)

Suicidal ideation		Suicidal intent	
Current plan		Risk to others	

4. LLCC assessment and management plan

Client name: ....

DOB: ....

Address: ....

....

Phone: ....

Next of kin: ....

....

Referral details: ....

....

Other: ....

....

Current concerns (timeframe and current stressors): ....

....

....

....

....

....

....

....

....

Relevant past history (past similar issues, previous counselling, relevant past medical history, mental health history): ....

....

....

....

....

....

....

....

....

Medication (prescribed or OTC): ....

....

Substance use (tobacco, alcohol, illicit drugs): ....

....

....

Personal and social history (use genogram; place of birth/culture; growing-up years
— primary school, friendships and interests; experience of high school/adolescence;
important family events; grief or trauma; adulthood — work/education, living
arrangements, interests and leisure activities; relationship history with family, work
colleagues, friends and partner relationships (present, past, same sex):

....

....

....

....

....

....

....

....

....

....

....

....

....

....

Explore risk factors (e.g. family history of mental health issues, recent stresses or
traumas): ....

....

....

....

....

....

....

Protective factors (e.g. past coping skills, positive social support, employment or financial stability): ....

....

....

....

....

....

Strategies or therapies that have been helpful previously to the client:

....

....

Any other areas relevant areas: ....

....

ASSESSMENT TOOLS

See K10/DASS etc.

HEADSS assessment tool:

    H = home

    E = education, employment, eating and exercise

    A = activities, hobbies and peer relationships

    D = drug use

    S = sexual activity and sexuality

    S = suicide, depression and mental health, safety/risk

RESULTS

Formulation

The 5Ps: presenting issues, precipitating, predisposing, perpetuating and protective factors for the issues:

Biological, psychological, social, cultural and spiritual (BPSCS): holistic in nature.

    1. Biological
- genetic factors (family history of illness), drug and alcohol use, medical illness and effects of medical
- treatments, including medication.

    2. Psychological:
- attachment style

■ temperament or the manner in which an individual responds to their environment (e.g. avoiding harm, responding to interpersonal relationships with vigilance, behaving impulsively or being dependent, seeking approval)
■ cognitive or thinking style
■ psychological coping mechanisms.

3. Social: available support, recent stressors, employment.
4. Cultural: range of cultural influences, plus experiences of the individual or past generations, such as trauma or displacement.
5. Spiritual: influences growing up or current influences.

MANAGEMENT PLAN

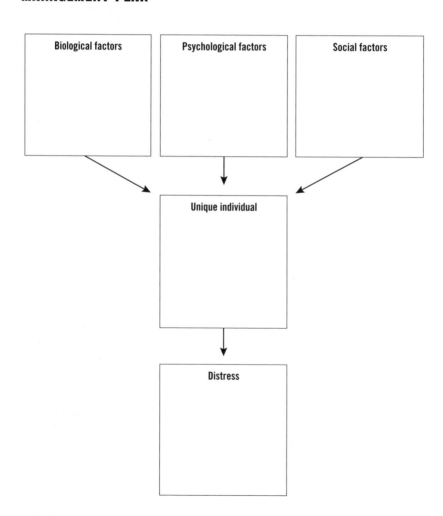

Client needs/issues/ problems (prioritized)	Goals	Therapies/ strategies

RELAPSE PREVENTION PLAN

Early warning symptoms and signs
1.
2.
3.
4.
5.

Possible high-risk situations for me
1.
2.
3.
How to cope with high-risk situations:

Emergency plan for relapse

5. Life domains and values

Life domain	'What is important to you/what do you value in this domain?'	'Is there a gap between what is currently happening and what you value?'
Family and friends		
Romance/intimate relationships		
Health and your body		
Education and personal development		
Work and finance		
Leisure (e.g. hobbies, relaxation time)		
Citizenship, community life (e.g. helping a neighbour, volunteering)		
Environment or nature		
Spirituality		

6. Graded exposure program

Factor/scenario	Anxiety (0–10)	Graded exposure steps

7. Managing negative thinking

Date/ time	What are you doing?	What are you thinking?	How do you feel?	Any unhelpful thinking patterns?	More helpful thoughts	How do you feel/ how are you now?

8. Interpersonal inventory

A review of current and past important relationships. Include:
- person's name, relationship with client, and age
- frequency of contact, shared activities, expectations (fulfilled or not)
- satisfactory or unsatisfactory aspects of relationship (concrete examples)
- ways client would like the relationship to change (including changing own or other's behaviour).

<table>
<tr><td></td><td></td></tr>
<tr><td></td><td></td></tr>
</table>

9. Mood diary

	Day 1	Day 2	Day 3	Day 4	Day 5	Day 6	Day 7
Mood (morning) Mood (evening) (0-10)							
Sleep							
Other (e.g. events, activities)							

10. Mood graph

Day/ Mood score	1	2	3	4	5	6	7	8	9	10	11	12	13	14
10														
9														
8														
7														
6														
5														
4														
3														
2														
1														
0														

11. Grief map[3]

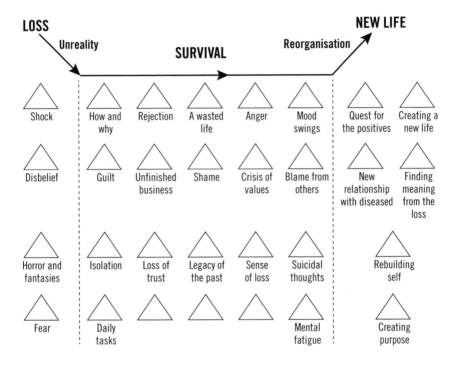

12. IPT conflict grid

Exploring interpersonal disputes	General statement	Specific incident
Content	1. Describe incident:	3. Gather more information:
Effect	2. Describe the effect:	4. Clarify effect further:

13. Self-care assessment[4]

The following worksheet for assessing self-care is not exhaustive, merely suggestive. Feel free to add areas of self-care that are relevant for you and rate yourself on how often and how well you are taking care of yourself these days. When you are finished, look for patterns in your responses. *Are you more active in some areas of self-care but ignore others? Are there items on the list that make you think, 'I would never do that'?* Listen to your inner responses, your internal dialogue about self-care and making yourself a priority. Take particular note of anything you would like to include more in your life.

Rate the following areas according to how well you think you are doing:

3 = I do this well (e.g. frequently)

2 = I do this okay (e.g. occasionally)

1 = I barely or rarely do this

0 = I never do this

? = This has never occurred to me

PHYSICAL SELF-CARE

- Eat regularly (e.g. breakfast, lunch, and dinner)
- Eat healthily
- Exercise
- Get regular medical care for prevention
- Get medical care when needed
- Take time off when sick
- Get massages
- Dance, swim, walk, run, play sports, sing or do some other fun physical activity
- Take time to be sexual — with myself, with a partner
- Get enough sleep
- Wear clothes I like
- Take vacations
- Other:

PSYCHOLOGICAL SELF-CARE

- Take day trips or mini-vacations
- Make time away from telephones, email and the internet
- Make time for self-reflection
- Notice my inner-experience — listen to my thoughts, beliefs, attitudes, feelings

- Have my own personal psychotherapy
- Write in a journal
- Read literature that is unrelated to work
- Do something at which I am not expert or in charge
- Attend to minimizing stress in my life
- Engage my intelligence in a new area e.g. go to an art show, sports event, theatre
- Be curious
- Say no to extra responsibilities sometimes
- Other:

EMOTIONAL SELF-CARE

- Spend time with others whose company I enjoy
- Stay in contact with important people in my life
- Give myself affirmations, praise myself
- Love myself
- Re-read favourite books, re-view favourite movies
- Identify comforting activities, objects, people, places, and seek them out
- Allow myself to cry
- Find things that make me laugh
- Express my outrage in social action, letters, donations, marches, protests
- Other:

SPIRITUAL SELF-CARE

- Make time for reflection
- Spend time in nature
- Find a spiritual connection or community
- Be open to inspiration
- Cherish my optimism and hope
- Be aware of non-material aspects of life
- Try at times not to be in charge or the expert
- Be open to not knowing
- Identify what is meaningful to me and notice its place in my life
- Meditate
- Pray
- Sing
- Have experiences of awe
- Contribute to causes in which I believe
- Read inspirational literature or listen to inspirational talks, music
- Other:

RELATIONSHIP SELF-CARE

- Schedule regular dates with my partner or spouse
- Schedule regular activities with my children
- Make time to see friends
- Call, check on or see my relatives
- Spend time with my companion animals
- Stay in contact with faraway friends
- Make time to reply to personal emails and letters; send holiday cards
- Allow others to do things for me
- Enlarge my social circle
- Ask for help when I need it
- Share a fear, hope or secret with someone I trust
- Other:

WORKPLACE OR PROFESSIONAL SELF-CARE

- Take a break during the work day (e.g. lunch)
- Take time to chat with co-workers
- Make quiet time to complete tasks
- Identify projects or tasks that are exciting and rewarding
- Set limits with clients and colleagues
- Balance my caseload so that no one day or part of a day is 'too much'
- Arrange work space so it is comfortable and comforting
- Get regular supervision or consultation
- Negotiate for my needs (benefits, pay rise)
- Have a peer support group
- Develop a non-trauma area of professional interest (if relevant)

OVERALL BALANCE

- Strive for balance within my work life and work day
- Strive for balance among work, family, relationships, play and rest

OTHER AREAS OF SELF-CARE THAT ARE RELEVANT TO YOU

-
-
-

Once you have completed the assessment, go back over it and reflect on your scores. Are there aspects you wish to continue with or change? Make a note of these.

Acknowledgments

This book would not have been possible without the support and education I have gained throughout my career from various colleagues, including Dr Michele Murphy. Several enthusiastic research assistants, Alyce Mayman, Greta Barrett and Charlotte Kelso, have also provided great help in relation to research for the book. Thanks also to Lauren Rauda, for kindly helping with the diagrams in the book and doing such a wonderful job. I would also like to thank my practice staff for coping with my preoccupation with writing, as well as family and friends, who supported me even though I became pretty unavailable to them for a time to finish the book! And a very special thanks to my clients who have been my teachers over the years.

Endnotes

Introduction

1. Howell, C. and Murphy, M. 2011, *Release Your Worries: A guide to letting go of stress and anxiety*, Exisle Publishing, New South Wales, p. 53.

Chapter 1

1. 'Caring' defintion, retrieved from www. oxforddictionaries.com

2. Psychotherapy and Counselling Federation of Australia, 2013, 'Counselling and psychotherapy' definition, retrieved from www.pacfa.org.au/practitioner-resources/ counselling-psychotherapy-definitions/

3. Yalom, I.D. 2002, *The Gift of Therapy: An open letter to a new generation of therapists and their patients*, California: HarperCollins, California, p. 6.

4. Horgan, D. 2015, 'Depression: What to talk about — a practical guide', Paper presented at the Health Matters: National General Practitioner Meeting, Sydney, 21–22 March 2015.

5. Corey, G. 1991, *Theory and Practice of Counseling and Psychotherapy* (4th ed.), Brooks/ Cole, California.

6. Egan, G. 2007, *The Skilled Helper: A problem-management and opportunity-development approach to helping* (8th ed.), Brooks/Cole, California.

7. Hutchinson, D. 2015, *The Essential Counsellor: Process, skills and techniques* (3rd ed.), Sage, Los Angeles.

8. Corey, G. 1991, op. cit., p. 210.

9. Corey, G. 2013,. *Theory and Practice of Counseling and Psychotherapy* (9th ed.), Cengage Learning, California, p. 177.

10. Corey, G. 1991, op. cit., p. 204.

11. ibid., p. 213–4.

12. University College London, Division of Psychology and Language Sciences. n.d., 'Ability to foster and maintain a good therapeutic alliance, and to grasp the client's perspective and "world view",' retrieved from http://www.ucl.ac.uk/clinical-psychology/ CORE/Psychodynamic_Competences/ Generic_Therapeutic_Competences/ Therapeutic_Alliance.pdf

13. Hutchinson, D., op. cit., p. 19.

14. Corey, G. 1991, op. cit., p. 115.

15. Dr Dot, 2008, 'Transferance and counter-transference', retrieved from http:// www.clinpsy.org.uk/forum/viewtopic. php?t=1979

16. ibid.

17. Hutchinson, D., op. cit., p. 28.

18. ibid.

19. ibid., p 92.

20. Marks-Tarlow, T. 2012, *Clinical Intuition in Psychotherapy: The neurobiology of embodied response*, W.W. Norton and Company, New York, p. viii.

21. Hutchinson, D., op. cit., p. 136.

22. Myers, D.G. 2002, *Intuition: Its powers and perils*, Yale University Press, London, p. 18.

23. Marks-Tarlow, T., op. cit., p. 3.

24. ibid., p. 42.

25. ibid., p. 11.

26. ibid., p. 56.

27. Corey, G. 2013, op. cit., p. 466.

28. ibid.

29. Lazarus, A. 2000,. 'Multimodal Therapy', in R.J. Corsini and D. Wedding (eds), *Current Psychotherapies*, Brooks/Cole, California, p. 342.

30. Dryden, W. and Mytton, J. 1999,. *Four Approaches to Counselling and Psychotherapy*, Routledge, London, p. 135.

31. Corey, G. 2013, op. cit., p. 271.

32. Palmer, S. (ed.) 2002, *Multicultural Counselling*, Sage Publications, London, p. 11.

33. ibid., p. 35.

34. ibid., p. 59.

35. ibid., p. 148.
36. Corey, G. 2013, op. cit., p. 363.
37. ibid., p. 373.
38. ibid., p. 369.

Chapter 2

1. Egan, G., op. cit., p. 68.
2. McGoldrick, M., Gerson, R. and Petry, S. 2008, *Genograms in Family Assessment*, W.W. Norton and Company, London, p. 2.
3. Galvin, K. 2015, 'Genograms: Constructing and interpreting interaction patterns', retrieved from http://genograms.org/symbols/
4. Krasucki, C. 1999, 'The FEAR: A rapid screening instrument for Generalised Anxiety in elderly primary care attenders', *International Journal of Geriatric Psychiatry*, 14, pp. 16–68.
5. Kessler, R.C., Andrews, G., Colpe, E. et al. 2002, 'Short screening scales to monitor population prevalences and trends in non-specific psychological distress', *Psychological Medicine*, 32, pp. 956–9.
6. Anderson, I. Michalak, E. et al., 2002, 'Depression in primary care: Tools for screening, diagnosis, and measuring response to treatment. *BCMJ*, 44(8), pp. 415–19.
7. Lovibond, S.H. and Lovibond, P.F. 1995, *Manual for the Depression Anxiety Stress Scales* (2nd ed.), Psychology Foundation, Sydney.
8. Cohen, E., MacKenzie, R.G., and Yates, G.L. 1991, 'HEADSS, a psychosocial risk assessment instrument: Implications for designing effective intervention programs for runaway youth', *Journal of Adolescent Health*, 12 7, pp. 539–44.
9. Sturney, P. (ed.) 2009, *Clinical Case Formulation: Varieties of approaches*, Wiley-Blackwell, United Kingdom, p. 145.
10. CALT Learning Support, 2015, 21 Feb 2007, 'Formulation example', retrieved from http://www.monash.edu.au/lls/llonline/writing/medicine/psychology/6.1.xml
11. Committee for Examinations, 2004, 'RANZCP clinical examinations formulation guidelines for trainees', retrieved from http://www.psychtraining.org/RANZCP-Formulations-Guide.pdf
12. Adapted from: Weissman, M.M., Markowitz, J. and Klerman, G. 2007, *Clinicians' Quick Guide to Interpersonal Psychotherapy*, Oxford University Press, United Kingdom.
13. Howell, C. and Murphy, M., op. cit., p. 43.
14. Harris, R. 2009a, *ACT Made Simple: An easy-to-read primer on Acceptance and Committment Therapy*, Harbinger Publications, Oakland USA.
15. Howell, C. and Murphy, M., op. cit., p. 44.
16. Adapted from R. Harris 2009a.
17. Howell, C. 2010, *Keeping the Blues Away: The ten-step guide to reducing the relapse of depression*, Radcliffe Publishing, Milton Keynes, p. 123.

Chapter 3

1. Grant, J. and Cadell, S. 2009, 'Power, pathological worldviews and the strengths perspective in social work', *Families in Society*, 90 40 , pp. 425–30.
2. Scerra, N. 2011, 'Strengths-based Practice: The evidence. A discussion paper', Social Justice Unit, UnitingCare Children, Young People and Families, p. 4.
3. Corey, 2013, ibid., p. 145.
4. ibid., p. 146.
5. ibid., p. 143.
6. Holmes, J. 1993, *John Bowlby and Attachment Theory*, Routledge, New York, p. 61.
7. ibid., p. 103.
8. Lazarus, A. op. cit., p. 342.
9. Harris, R. 2009a, op. cit., p. 8.
10. Siegel, D.J. 2007, *The Mindful Brain: Reflection and attunement in the cultivation of wellbeing*, W.W. Norton and Company, New York, p. 31.
11. Harris, R. 2013, 'Mindfulness', retrieved from http://www.actmindfully.com.au
12. Neff, K. 2003, 'Self-compassion: An alternative conceptualisation of a healthy attitude toward oneself', *Self and Identity*, 2, p. 86.
13. Sheldon, K. and King, L. 2001, 'Why Positive Psychology is necessary', *American Psychologist*, 54 3, p. 216.
14. Compton, W. 2005, *An Introduction to Positive Psychology*, Wadsworth, California, p. 8.
15. Fredrickson, B. 2009, *Positivity: Groundbreaking research to release your inner optimist and thrive*, OneWorld Publications, London, pp. 9–11.
16. Seligman, M. 2011, *Flourish: A visionary new understanding of happiness and wellbeing*, Random House Australia, Sydney.

17. Noonan, W.C. and Moyers, T.B. 1997, 'Motivational Interviewing: A review', *Journal of Substance Misuse*, 2, p. 8.

18. ibid., pp. 8–16.

19. Miller, W. R. and Rollnick, S. 2002,. *Motivational Interviewing: Preparing people for change* (2nd ed.), Guilford Press, New York.

20. Noonan and Moyers, op. cit.

21. 'Bathe technique', 2015, retrieved from http://www.fpnotebook.com/psych/exam/BthTchnq.htm

22. Sharf, R. 2008, *Theories of Psychotherapy and Counselling: Concepts and cases* (4th ed.), Brooks/Cole, California.

23. ibid., p. 482.

24. Beck Institute for Cognitive Behavior Therapy. n.d., 'History of Cognitive Therapy', retrieved from http://www.beckinstitute.org/history-of-cbt/

25. Howell, C. 2010, op. cit., p. 69.

26. ibid., p. 74.

27. Segal, Z., Williams, J.M.G. and Teasdale, J.D. 2002, *Mindfulness-based Cognitive Therapy for Depression: A new approach to preventing relapse*, Guilford Press, New York, p. 27.

28. Felder, J.N., Dimidijan, S. and Segal, Z. 2012, 'Collaboration in Mindfulness-based Cognitive Therapy', *Journal of Clinical Psychology*, 68 2 , p. 180.

29. Manicavasagar, V., Perich, T. and Parker, G. 2012, 'Cognitive predictors of change in Cognitive Behavioural Therapy and Mindfulness-based Cognitive Therapy for depression', *Behavioural and Cognitive Psychotherapy*, 40, p. 227.

30. Linehan, M.M. 1993, as cited in Eisendrath, S., Chartier, M. and McLane, M. 2010, 'Adapting Mindfulness-based Cognitive Therapy for Treatment-Resistant Depression', *Cognitive and Behavioural Practice*, 18 10, p. 362.

31. Harris, R. 2009a, op. cit., p. 2.

32. Howell, C. and Murphy, M., p 162 .

33. Eifert, G. and Forsyth, J. 2005, *Acceptance and Commitment Therapy for Anxiety Disorders: A practitioner's treatment guide to using mindfulness, acceptance and values-based behaviour change strategies*, New Harbinger Publications, California, p. 16.

34. Harris, R., 2009a, op. cit., p. 8.

35. ibid.

36. Klerman, G., Weissman, M.M. et al. 1999, *Interpersonal Psychotherapy of Depression: A brief, focused, specific strategy*, Jason Aronson, London, p. 73.

37. Stuart, S. and Robertson, M. 2003, *Interpersonal Psychotherapy: A clinician's guide*, Hodder Arnold, London, p. 93.

38. White, C. and Denborough, D. (eds) 1998, *Introducing Narrative Therapy: A collection of practice-based writings*, Dulwich Centre Publications, Adelaide, p. 3.

39. Howell, C. and Murphy, M., op. cit., p. 181.

40. White, C. and Denborough, D., op. cit., p. 73.

41. Andrews, J. and Clark, D. 1996, 'In the case of a depressed woman: Solution-focused or Narrative Therapy approaches?', *The Family Journal*, 4, p. 243.

42. Launer, J. 2002, *Narrative-based Primary Care*, Radcliffe Publishing, Milton Keynes, p. 35.

43. White, M. 1995, 'Naming abuse and breaking from its effects', *Re-authoring Lives: Interviews and essays*, Dulwich Centre Publications, Adelaide, pp. 82–111.

44. White, M. 2007 . *Maps of Narrative Practice*, W.W. Norton and Company, New York, p. 61.

45. Launer, J., op. cit., p. 35.

46. Corey, G. 2013, op. cit., p. 417.

47. Seligman, M., op. cit., p. 40.

48. Hammond, D. 1988, *Hypnotic Induction and Suggestion: An introductory manual*, American Society of Clinical Hypnosis, Illinois, p. 263.

49. Hammond, D. 2010, 'Hypnosis in the treatment of anxiety- and stress-related disorders', *Expert Review of Neurotherapeutics*, 10 2 , pp. 263–73.

50. Montgomery, G.H., DuHamel, K.N.,and Redd, W.H. 2000, 'A meta-analysis of hypnotically induced analgesia: How effective is hypnosis?', *International Journal of Clinical and Experimental Hypnosis*, 48, pp. 138, 263.

51. Chapman, A. 2014, *Integrating Clinical Hypnosis and CBT: Treating depression, anxiety and fears*, Springer, New York.

52. Owen, N. 2001, *The Magic of Metaphor: 77 stories for teachers, trainers and thinkers*, Crown House, Wales, p. 5.

53. Krasner, M.A. 2002, *The Wizard Within: The Krasner method of hypnotherapy*, American

Board of Hypnotherapy Press, California, p. 92.

54. Owen, N. op. cit., p. xv.

55. Burns, G.W. 2007, *Healing With Stories: Your casebook collection for using therapeutic metaphors'*, Wiley, New Jersey, p. 19.

56. Owen, N. 2005, *More Magic of Metaphor: Stories for leaders, influencers and motivators*, Crown House, Wales.

57. Corey, 2013, op. cit., p. 189.

58. Anderson, L., Lewis, G. and Araya, R. et al. 2005, 'Self-help books for depression: How can practicioners and patients make the right choice?' *British Journal of General Practice*, 55 514 , pp. 387–92.

59. Cuijpers, P. 1997, 'Bibliotherapy in unipolar depression: A meta-analysis', *Journal of Behavior Therapy and Experimental Psychiatry'*, 28 2 , pp. 139–47.

60. Cuijpers, P., van Straten, A. and Smit, F. 2006, 'Psychological treatment of late-life depression: A meta-analysis of randomized controlled trials', *International Journal of Geriatric Psychiatry*, 21, pp. 1139–49.

61. Gregory, R.J., Schwer Canning, S., Lee, T.W. and Wise, J.C. 2004, 'Cognitive bibliotherapy for depression: A meta-analysis', *Professional Psychology: Research and Practice*, 35 3 , pp. 275–80.

62. Brewster, L. 2008, 'The reading remedy: Bibliotherapy in practice', *Australasian Public Libraries and Information Services*, 21 4, retrieved from https://www.questia.com/read/1G1-190747229/the-reading-remedy-bibliotherapy-in-practice

63. Usher, T.M. 2015, 'The Reader's View of Using Bibliotherapy to Cope with Depression', PhD thesis.

64. Russell, D.H. and Shrodes, C. 1950, 'Contributions of research in bibliotherapy to the language-arts program', *The School Review*, 58 6 , pp. 335–42.

65. Cohen, L.J. 1994, 'The experience of therapeutic reading', *Western Journal of Nursing Research*, 16 4, pp. 426.

66. Cilliers, J.I. 1983, 'Biblioterapie vir alkoholiste en dwelmafhanklikes', *Humanitas: Journal for Research in the Human Sciences*, 9 2 , pp. 195–209.

67. Usher, T.M., op. cit.

68. Barak, A., Klein, B. and Proudfoot, J.G. 2009, 'Defining internet-supported therapeutic interventions', *Annals of Behavioural Medicine*, 38 1, pp. 4–17.

69. Reynolds, J., Griffiths, K.M., Cunningham, J.A., Bennett, K. and Bennett, A. 2015, 'Clinical practice models for the use of e-mental health resources in primary health care by health professionals and peer workers: A conceptual framework', *JMIR Mental Health*, 2 1, p. e6.

70. Royal Australian College of General Practitioners 2015, 'e-Mental health: A guide for GPs' p. 8.

71. Moock, J. 2014, 'Support from the internet for individuals with mental disorders: Advantages and disadvantages of e-mental health service delivery', *Front Public Health*, 2, 65.

72. Handbook of Non Drug Interventions HANDI Project Team 2013, 'Internet-based Cognitive Behaviour Therapy for depression and anxiety', *Australian Family Physician*, 42 11, pp. 803–4.

73. Hoifodt, R.S., Strom, C., Kolstrup, N., Eisemann, M. and Waterloo, K. 2011, 'Effectiveness of Cognitive Behavioural Therapy in primary health care: A review', *Family Practicioner*, 28 5, pp. 489–504.

74. National Institute for Health and Clinical Excellence 2009, *Depression in Adults: The treatment and management of depression in adults.* NICE, London.

75. Royal Australian College of General Practitioners 2015, 'e-Mental health: A guide for GPs', RACGP, Mebourne.

Chapter 4

1. Howell, C. 2010, op. cit., pp. 32–4.

2. headspace 2015, 'Tips for a healthy headspace', retrieved from http://headspace.org.au/get-info/tips-for-a-healthy-headspace

3. Better Health Channel 2015a, 'Sleep', retrieved from http://www.betterhealth.vic.gov.au/bhcv2/bhcarticles.nsf/pages/Sleep?open

4. Division of Sleep Medicine 2008, 'You and your biological clock', retrieved from http://healthysleep.med.harvard.edu/healthy/getting/bio-clock

5. Sleepdex 2014, 'Circadian cycles and sleep', retrieved from http://www.sleepdex.

org/circadian2.htm

6. Better Health Channel, 2015a, op.c it.
7. Smith, M., Robinson, L. and Segal, R. 2015, 'The importance of deep sleep and REM sleep', retrieved from http://www.helpguide.org/articles/sleep/how-much-sleep-do-you-need.htm
8. ibid.
9. Better Health Channel, 2015a, op. cit.
10. ibid.
11. ibid.
12. Division of Sleep Medicine 2008a, 'Why sleep matters: Consequences of insufficient sleep', retrieved from http://healthysleep.med.harvard.edu/healthy/matters
13. Nicholas, M., Molloy, A., Tonkin, L. and Beeston, L. 2004, *Manage Your Pain: Practical and positive ways of adapting to chronic pain*, ABC Books, Sydney, p. 161.
14. Howell, C. 2010, op. cit., p. 160.
15. Better Health Channel. 2015b, 'Sleep hygiene', retrieved from http://www.betterhealth.vic.gov.au/bhcv2/bhcarticles.nsf/pages/Sleep_hygiene.
16. Howell, C. 2010, op. cit.
17. Howell, C. and Murphy, M., op. cit.
18. Cline, J. 2009, 'Cognitive Behavioural Therapy for insomnia Part 4: Sleep restriction', *Psychology Today*, 13 July.
19. Alman, B.M. and Lambrou, P. 2013, *Self-hypnosis: The complete manual for health and self-change*, Brunner/Mazel, Philadelphia.
20. Hunter, M. 1994, *Creative Scripts for Hypnotherapy*, Routledge, New York.

Chapter 5

1. Howell, C. and Murphy, M., op. cit.
2. Howell, C. 2010, op. cit.
3. Howell, C. and Murphy, M., op. cit.
4. Eifert, G. and Forsyth, J., op. cit., p. 45.
5. American Psychiatric Association 2013, *Diagnostic and Statistical Manual of Mental Disorders* (5th ed.) American Psychiatric Publishing, Virginia.
6. Howell, C. and Murphy, M., op. cit., pp. 13–14.
7. ibid., p. 14.
8. ibid., p. 20.
9. Wells, A. 1997, *Cognitive Therapy of Anxiety Disorders: A practice manual and conceptual guide*,

Wiley, West Sussuex..

10. Howell, C. and Murphy, M., op. cit., p. 67.
11. ibid., p. 61.
12. Hassed, C. 2002, *Know Thyself: The stress relief program*, Michelle Anderson Publishing, Melbourne, p. 50.
13. O'Donoghue, M. 2009, 'Teaching meditation 1: Concentration on the breath', *Journal of the Australian and New Zealand Student Services Association*, 33, 62.
14. Howell, C. and Murphy, M., op. cit.
15. Howell, C. 2013, *Intuition: Unlock the power!* Exisle Publishing, New South Wales, p. 62.
16. Wells, A., op. cit.
17. ibid.
18. Howell, C. and Murphy, M., op. cit., p. 140.
19. Howell, C. 2010, op. cit., p. 46.
20. ibid., p. 46.
21. ibid., p. 47.
22. Walsh, C. 2006, 'The "just worrying" labelling technique', retrieved from http://www.mindfulness.org.au/the-just-worrying-labelling-technique/
23. Harris, R. 2009a, op. cit., p. 53.
24. ibid., p. 11.
25. Howell, C. and Murphy, M., op. cit., p. 167.
26. ibid., p. 80.
27. ibid., p. 165.
28. Harris, R. 2007, op. cit., p. 95.
29. ibid.
30. Howell, C. and Murphy, M., op. cit., p. 167.
31. ibid., p. 168.
32. ibid., p. 169.
33. ibid., p. 170.
34. ibid., p. 172.
35. Harris, R. 2009a, op. cit., p. 150.
36. Harris, R. 2010, *The Confidence Gap*, Penguin, Melbourne, p. 130.
37. White, M. 2007, op. cit.
38. White, M. 1995, op. cit.
39. Howell, C. and Murphy, M., op. cit., p. 189, based on Linell, S. and Cora, D. 1993, *Discoveries: A group resource guide for women who have been sexually abused in childhood*, Dympna House Publications, Sydney.
40. Linley, P.A., Nielsen, K.M., Wood, A.M., Gillett, R. and Biswas-Diener, R. 2010, 'Using signature strengths in pursuit of goals: Effects on goal progress, need satisfaction, and wellbeing, and implications

for coaching psychologists', *International Coaching Psychology Review*, 5 1 , p. 59.

41. Lyubomirsky, S. 2007, *The How of Happiness: A practical guide to getting the life you want*, Sphere, London.

42. ibid., p. 95.

43. Dowrick, S. 2007, *Creative Journal Writing:Tthe art and heart of reflection*, Allen & Unwin, Sydney.

44. Compton, W., op. cit., p. 166.

45. Masten, A.S., Best, K.M. and Garmezy, N. 1990, 'Resilience and development: Contributions from the study of children who overcome adversity', *Development and Psychopathology*, 2 4 , pp. 425–44.

46. Fredrickson, B., op. cit.

47. Siebert, A. 2005, *The Resiliency Advantage: Master change, thrive under pressure and bounce back from setbacks*, Berrett-Koehler Publications, California.

Chapter 6

1. Howell, C., op. cit., p. 19.

2. Klerman, G., Weissman, M.M. et al., op. cit., p. 17.

3. Howell, C., op. cit., p. 29.

4. Howell, C., op. cit., p. 30.

5. Lawlor, D. and Hopker, S. 2001, 'The effectiveness of exercise as an intervention in the management of depression: Systematic review and meta-regression analysis of randomised clinical trials', *British Medical Journal*, 322, p. 763.

6. Howell, C., op. cit., p. 45.

7. Sharf, R., op. cit., p. 482.

8. Howell, C., op. cit., p. 64.

9. ibid., p. 100.

10. ibid., p. 105.

11. ibid., p. 64.

12. ibid., p. 69.

13. ibid., p. 73.

14. Greenberger, D. and Padesky, C. 2016, *Mind Over Mood: Change how you feel by changing the way you think*, (2nd ed.), Guilford Press, New York, p. 156.

15. Centre for Clinical Interventions, 2008, 'Perfectionism in perspective', retrieved from http://www.cci.health.wa.gov.au/resources/infopax.cfm?Info_ID=52

16. Howell, C., op. cit., p. 75.

17. Howell, C. and Murphy, M., op. cit., p. 143–7.

18. Segal, Z., Williams, J.M.G. and Teasdale, J.D. 2002, *Mindfulness-based Cognitive Therapy for Depression: A new approach to preventing relapse*, Guilford Press, New York.

19. Kuyken, W., Byford, S., Taylor, R.S. et al. 2008, 'Mindfulness-based Cognitive Therapy to prevent relapse in recurrent depression', *Journal of Consulting and Clinical Psychology*, 76, p. 64.

20. Manicavasagar, V., Perich, T. and Parker, G. 2012, 'Cognitive predictors of change in Cognitive Behavioural Therapy and Mindfulness-based Cognitive Therapy for depression', *Behavioural and Cognitive Psychotherapy*, 40, pp. 227–232

21. Segal, Z., Williams, J.M.G. and Teasdale, J.D., op. cit.

22. ibid., p. 81.

23. Zettle, R.D. 2007, *ACT for Depression: A clinician's guide to using Acceptance and Commitment Therapy in treating depression*, New Harbinger Publications, California, p. 38–40.

24. Harris, R. 2009a, op. cit., p. 192.

25. ibid., p. 93.

26. ibid., p. 149.

27. Klerman, G., Weissman, M.M. et al., op. cit., p. 17.

28. ibid., p. 53.

29. ibid., p. 55–61.

30. ibid., p. 48–9.

31. Howell, C., op. cit., p. 116.

32. ibid., p. 109.

33. ibid., p. 94.

34. ibid., p. 110.

35. ibid.

36. Page, A. and Page, C. 1996, *Assert Yourself! How to resolve conflict and say what you mean without being passive or aggressive*, Gore and Osment, Sydney.

37. Howell, C., op. cit., p. 112.

38. ibid.

39. O'Connor, R. 2001, *Active Treatment of Depression*, Norton, New York, p. 112.

40. Howell, C. 2013, op. cit., p. 47.

41. Moran, C. 2003, 'Beyond content: Does humor help coping?', *Disability Quarterly*, 3, 5.

42. Zournani, M. 2002, *Hope: New philosophies for*

change, Pluto Press, Sydney, p. 14.

43. Marsden, V. 2012, 'Holding on tight: Creative ways to hold on to hope between counselling sessions', *Explorations: An e-journal of narrative practice*, 4 , p. 75, retrieved from http://dulwichcentre.com.au/explorations-2012-1-victoria-marsden.pdf

44. Anderson, L., Lewis, G., Araya, R. et al. 2005, 'Self-help books for depression: How can practicioners and patients make the right choice?' *British Journal of General Practice*, 55 514, pp. 387–392.

45. Cuijpers, P., op. cit.

46. Cuijpers, P., van Straten, A. and Smit, F., op. cit.

47. Gregory, R.J., Schwer Canning, S., Lee, T.W. and Wise, J.C., op. cit.

48. Ahmadipour, T., Avand, F. and Mo'menpour, S. 2012, 'Bibliotherapy on depressed university students: A case study', *Studies in Literature and Language*, 4 2, pp. 49–57 .

Chapter 7

1. Petracek, L.J. 2004, *The Anger Workbook for Women*, New Harbinger Publications, California, p. 35.

2. ibid., p.37 .

3. ibid., p. 25.

4. ibid., p. 2.

5. Harris, R. 2009b, op. cit., p. 131.

6. Gottman, J.M. and Silver, N. 2007, *The Seven Principles for Making Marriage Work*, Orion, London, p. 29.

7. ibid., p. 87.

8. Schuldt, W. 2015, 'Fair fighting rules', retrieved from http://www.therapistaid.com/therapy-worksheets/relationships/none

Chapter 8

1. Brown, B. 2010, *The Gifts of Imperfection: Let go of who you think you're supposed to be and embrace who you are*, Hazelden Publishing, Minnesota, p. 39.

2. Brown, B. 2012, *Daring Greatly: How the courage to be vulnerable transforms the way we live, love, parent, and lead*, Penguin, NewYork, p. 68.

3. Brown, B. 2010, op. cit., p. 41.

4. ibid., p. 46.

5. Brown, B. 2012, p. 75.

6. ibid., p. 2.

7. ibid., p. 116.

8. Harris, R. 2009b, op. cit., p. 116.

Chapter 9

1. 'Change' definition, retrieved from http://www.oxforddictionaries.com

2. Nicholas, M., Molloy, A., Tonkin, L. and Beeston, L. 2004, op. cit., p. 90.

3. Sprague, R. 1984, 'The high cost of personal transitions', *Training and Development Journal*, pp. 61–63.

4. Smith, C.A. and Lazarus, R.S. 1990, 'Emotion and adaption' in L. A. Pervin, L.A. (ed.) *Handbook of Personality Theory and Research*, Guilford, New York.

5. White, M. 1995, op. cit.

6. Abu-Rayyan, N.M. 2009, 'Seasons of life: Ex-detainees reclaiming their lives', *International Journal of Narrative Therapy and Community Work*, 2, p. 28.

7. Turner, V. 1969, *The Ritual Process: Structure and anti-structure*, Aldine de Gruyter, New York.

8. Source: Abu-Rayyan, N.M., op. cit.

9. Schroder, D. 2005, *Little Windows Into Art Therapy: Small opening for beginning therapists*, Jessica Kingsley Publishers, London, p. 9.

10. Frederickson, B. 2001, 'The role of positive emotions in Positive Psychology: The broaden-and-build theory of positive emotions', American Psychologist, 56 3 , pp. 218–26.

11. Seligman, M., op. cit., p. 40.

Chapter 10

1. Barkway, P. 2013, *Psychology for Health Professionals*, Elsevier, Sydney.

2. Bull, M. 2009, 'Loss' in Barkway, P. (ed.), *Psychology for Health Professionals*, Elsevier, Sydney, p. 207.

3. Doka, K.J. 1989, *Disenfranchised Grief: Recognising hidden sorrow*, Lexington Books, England, p. 4.

4. Bull, M., op. cit., p. 204.

5. ibid., p. 206.

6. ibid., p. 203.

7. ibid., p. 212.

8. ibid.

9. ibid., p. 212–3.

10. ibid., p. 212.

11. ibid. p. 207.

12. Bowlby 1980, quoted in Bull, M. op. cit., p. 207.

13. Sanders, C.M. 1999, *Grief: The mourning after: Dealing with adult bereavement* (2nd ed.), Wiley, New York.

14. Bull, M., op. cit., p. 207.

15. ibid., p. 216.

16. Adapted from Bull, M. 2009.

17. Bull, M. 2009, p. 204.

18. Worden 2008 in in Bull, M. 2009.

19. ibid.

20. Bull, M. 2009, p. 210.

21. Neimeyer, R., Burke, L. et al. 2010, 'Grief therapy and the reconstruction of meaning: From principles to practice', *J Contemp Psychother*, 40 2, pp. 73–83.

22. Neimeyer, R.A. 2014, 'Robert Neimeyer Ph.D', retrieved from http://www.meaning.ca/conference/robert-neimeyer-phd/ .

23. Bull, M. op. cit., p. 210.

24. ibid., p. 211.

25. ibid., pp. 214–15.

26. ibid., p. 213.

27. Worden 2008 in Bull, M. 2009, p .214.

28. Neimeyer, R., Burke, L. et al. op. cit.

29. Clark, S. 2001, 'Mapping grief: An active approach to grief resolution', *Death Studies*, 25, pp. 531–48.

30. White, C. and Denborough, D. op. cit.

31. White, C. and Denborough D. 1988, *Introduction to Narrative Therapy: A collection of practice-based writings*, Dulwich Centre Publications, Adelaide, p. 29.

32. 'Memory boxes and alters', retrieved from http://www.recover-from-grief.com

33. Howell, C. 2010, p. 93.

34. Based on the work of Sheila Clark in Clark, S. 1995, *After Suicide: Help for the bereaved*, Hill of Content, Melbourne.

Chapter 11

1. Wade, D., Howard, A. et al. 2013, 'Early response to psychological trauma: What GPs can do', *Australian Family Physician*, 42 9, p. 610.

2. BC Provincial Mental Health and Substance Use Planning Council 2013, 'Trauma-informed practice guide', p. 9.

3. ibid., p. 6.

4. ibid., p. 7.

5. American Psychiatric Association, op. cit.

6. Briere, J. and Scott, C. 2012, *Principles of Trauma Therapy: A guide to symptoms, evaluation and treatment* (2nd ed.), Sage, Los Angeles.

7. ibid., p. 52.

8. Prins, A., Ouimette, P. et al. 2003, 'The primary care PTSD screen PC-PTSD: Development and operating characteristics', *Primary Care Psychiatry*, 9, pp. 9–14.

9. Hopper, E., Bassuk, E. and Olivet, J. 2010, 'Shelter from the storm: Trauma informed care in homelessness services settings', *The Open Health Services and Policy Jounral*, 3, p. 52.

10. Poole, N. and Greaves, L. 2012, *Becoming Trauma Informed*, Centre for Addiction and Mental Health, Toronto.

11. BC Provincial Mental Health and Substance Use Planning Council, op. cit., pp. 13–14.

12. ibid., p. 53.

13. ibid., p. 41.

14. Australian Centre for Post-traumatic Health 2013, 'Australian Guidelines for the Treatment of Adults with Acute Stress Disorder and Posttraumatic Disorder', NHMRC, Australian Government, p. 69.

15. BC Provincial Mental Health and Substance Use Planning Council, op. cit., p. 28.

16. Australian Centre for Post-traumatic Health, op. cit., p. 69–70.

17. Royal Australian College of General Practitioners, op. cit.

18. Australian Centre for Post-traumatic Health, op. cit.

19. Gonzalez-Prendos, A. and Resko, M, 2012, 'Cognitive Behaviour Therapy' in Ringel, S. and Brandell, J. (eds), *Trauma: Contemporary directions in theory, practice, and research*. Sage, Los Angeles, p. 17.

20. Harris, R. 2009a, op. cit., p. 11.

21. White, C. and Denborough, D., op. cit.

Chapter 12

1. Harris, R. 2009b, op. cit., p. 9.
2. R. Harris, 2009b, p. 14 .
3. Cassidy, J. and Shaver, P. 2008, *Handbook of Attachment Theory, Research, and Clincial Applciations*, Guilford Press, New York, p. 214.
4. ibid., p. 814.
5. ibid., p. 821.
6. ibid., p. 813.
7. Gottman, J.M. and Silver, N. 2007, *The Seven Principles for Making Marriage Work*, Orion, London, p. 22.
8. ibid., p. 83.
9. ibid., p. 25.
10. Harris, R. 2009b, p. 20.
11. ibid., p. 36.
12. ibid., p. 99.
13. ibid., p. 101.
14. ibid., p. 127.
15. ibid., p. 190.
16. ibid., p. 189.
17. ibid., p. 212.
18. Chapman, G. 2010, *The 5 Love Languages: The secret to love that lasts*, Northfield Publishing, Chicago, p. 23.
19. Gottman J.M. and Silver, N., op. cit., p. 79.
20. ibid., p. 93.
21. ibid., p. 48.
22. ibid., p. 57.
23. Harris, V.W. 2015, 'Nine important communication skills for every relationship', retrieved from http://www.edis.ifas.ufl.edu/m/ - publication?id=FY1277
24. Harris, R. 2009b, op. cit., p. 54.
25. ibid., p. 153.
26. Gottman, J.M. 1994, *Why Marriages Succeed or Fail: And how to make yours last*, Fireside, New York.
27. ibid.
28. Harris, R. 2009b, op. cit., p. 165.
29. ibid., p. 170.
30. ibid., p. 43.
31. Gottman J.M. and Silver, N., op. cit., p. 68.
32. ibid., p. 70.
33. ibid., p. 73.
34. Harris, R. 2009b, op. cit., p. 36.
35. ibid., p. 156.
36. Gottman J.M. and Silver, N., op. cit., p. 99.
37. ibid., p. 184.
38. Harris, R. 2009b, op. cit., p. 100.
39. Harris, R. 2009b, op. cit., p. 135.
40. ibid., p. 130.
41. ibid., p. 153.
42. Harris, R. 2009b, op. cit., p. 137.
43. Harris, R. 2009b, op. cit., p. 144.
44. ibid., p. 77.
45. Harris, R. 2009b, op. cit., p. 199.
46. Chapman, G., op. cit., p. 187.
47. Gottman J.M. and Silver, N., op. cit., p. 173.
48. ibid., p. 217.
49. Harris, R. 2009b, op. cit., p. 36.

Chapter 13

1. Howell, C. 2010, op. cit., p. 80.
2. Neff, K., op. cit., p. 86.
3. Harris, R. 2010, op. cit., p. 99.
4. ibid., p. 73.
5. Howell, C. 2010, op. cit., p. 81.
6. ibid., p. 65.
7. ibid., p. 82.
8. Harris, R. 2010, op. cit., p. 219.
9. ibid., p. 19.
10. ibid., p. 48.
11. ibid., p. 218.
12. ibid., p. 77.
13. Harris, R. 2009a, op. cit., p. 181.
14. Harris, R. 2010, op. cit., p. 159.
15. ibid., p. 197.
16. ibid., p. 237.
17. ibid p.239
18. ibid., p. 251.
19. Seligman, M., op. cit., p. 16.
20. Compton, W., op. cit., p. 48.
21. Linley, P.A., Nielsen, K.M., Wood, A.M., Gillett, R. and Biswas-Diener, R. 2010, 'Using signature strengths in pursuit of goals: Effects on goal progress, need satisfaction, and wellbeing, and implications for coaching psychologists', *International Coaching Psychology Review*, 5 1, p. 59.
22. ibid., p. 90.
23. ibid., p. 43.
24. Lyubomirsky, S., op. cit., p. 95.
25. Howell, C. 2013, op. cit., p. 130.
26. ibid., p. 132.

27. Retrieved from http://en.wikipedia.org/wiki/Milton_H._Erickson
28. Howell, C. 2013, op. cit., p. 162.
29. C. Howell, C. 2010, p. 133, based on Hammond, D. 1990, op. cit., p. 133.
30. Based on James, T. 2010, 'NLP practitioner training', The Tad James Company, USA.
31. Howell, C. 2013, op. cit., p. 164.

Chapter 14

1. Mitchell, J. 2015, 'What is crisis counselling', retrieved from http://www.acs.edu.au
2. ibid.
3. SQUARE 2006, 'Foundations for effective practice', p. 17.
4. Beyondblue2015, 'Suicide prevention program', retrieved from www.beyondblue.org.au/about-us/programs/mens-program/program-activities/suicide-prevention-program
5. Centers for Disease Control and Prevention, 'Suicide and self-inflicted injury', retrieved from http://www.cdc.gov/nchs/fastats/suicide.htm
6. Mental Health Foundation, 'Mental health statistics: suicide', retrieved from http://www.mentalhealth.org.uk/help-information/mental-health-statistics/suicide/
7. American Foundation for Suicide Prevention 2015, 'Suicide risk factors', retrieved from http://www.afsp.org
8. Chiles, J. and Strosahl, K. 2004, Clinical Manual for Assessment and Treatment of Suicidal Patients, American Psychiatric Publishing, Virginia, p. 69.
9. ibid., p.69.
10. American Foundation for Suicide Prevention, op. cit.
11. Chiles, J. and Strosahl, K., op. cit.
12. Beyondblue, op. cit.
13. SQUARE, op. cit., pp. 18–19.
14. ibid., p. 35.
15. ibid., p. 28.
16. Chiles, J. and Strosahl, K., op. cit., p. 69.
17. This assessment was written by Dr Cate Howell and Brian Williams, adapted from Sheehan, D., et al. 2000, 'The Mini International Neuropsychiatric Interview (MINI)'.
18. SQUARE, op. cit., p. 47.
19. Miller, I., Norman, W., Bishop, S. et al. 1991, 'Modified Scale for Suicidal Ideation'.
20. SQUARE, op. cit., p. 22.
21. Hagwood, J. and De Leo, D. 2015, 'Working with suicidal clients: Impacts on psychologists and the need for self-care', InPsych, 37.

Chapter 15

1. Compassion Fatigue Awareness Project 2013, 'What is compassion fatigue?' retrieved from http://www.compassionfatigue.org
2. Adults Surviving Child Abuse 2015, 'Vicarious traumatisation', retrieved from http://www.asca.org.au
3. ibid.
4. ibid.
5. Evans, A. 2015, 'Self-care for psychologists: lifeline's learnings', InPsych, pp. 14–15.
6. Neff, K., op. cit., p. 86.
7. Neff, K., op. cit.
8. C. Howell, C. 2013, op. cit., p. 132.

Appendix

1. Andrews, G. and Slade T. 2001, 'Interpreting scores on the K10', ANZ Journal of Public Health, 25, 6, pp. 494–7.
2. Adapted from Family Planning Queensland 2005, 'HEADSS adolescent health check', retrieved from https://www.som.uq.edu.au/media/418866/headds.pdf.
3. Source: Clark, S. 2001, 'Mapping grief: An active approach to grief resolution', Death Studies, 25, pp. 531–48.
4. Adapted from Saakvitne, K. and Pearlman, L. 1996, Transforming the Pain: A workbook on vicarious traumatisation, W.W. Norton and Company, New York.

Index